AF556800

ADVANCED
GERIATRIC MEDICINE
6

ADVANCED GERIATRIC MEDICINE 6

Edited by

F. I. Caird MA, DM, FRCP

David Cargill Professor of Geriatric Medicine, University of Glasgow

and

J. Grimley Evans MA, MD, DM, FRCP, FFCM

Professor of Geriatric Medicine, University of Oxford

WRIGHT

Bristol
1987

Published under the Wright imprint by
IOP Publishing Limited
Techno House, Redcliffe Way, Bristol BS1 6NX

British Library Cataloguing in Publication Data

Advanced geriatric medicine.
6
1. Geriatrics
I. Caird, F. I.,
II. Evans, John Grimley
618.97 RC952

ISBN 0-7236-0651-X

Typeset by
Bath Typesetting Ltd

Printed in Great Britain by
The Bath Press, Lower Bristol Road, Bath BA2 3BL

Preface

Geriatric medicine and its scientific base in medical gerontology move on apace. Indeed the image of the complete geriatrician who could claim expert status in all matters relating to the elderly has vanished in the information explosion. We are all subspecialists nowadays. This volume is a continuation of a series that aims to provide broadly ranging reviews of topics relevant to the care of elderly people for doctors with a variety of interests and experience. The mixture is of science and practical business, and the authorship includes both the new and the established.

F. I. Caird
J. Grimley Evans

Acknowledgements

This volume is one of a series to which the Cardiovascular Forum of Smith Kline & French Ltd has contributed generous financial support.

It is a pleasure to acknowledge Mrs M. Smith's secretarial skills and Mr Roy Baker's tolerance of editorial delays.

Contributors

D. B. Brock PhD
Chief, Biometry Office
National Institute on Aging, Bethesda, USA
The Changing Demography of the Elderly in the United States

J. A. Brody MD
Dean, School of Public Health
University of Illinois at Chicago, Chicago, USA
The Changing Demography of the Elderly in the United States

F. I. Caird MA DM FRCP
David Cargill Professor of Geriatric Medicine
University of Glasgow
Favourable Demographic Aspects of the Elderly for the Next 30 Years

D. M. Carter MD PhD
The Rockefeller University,
New York, USA
Modern Dressings for Leg Ulcers

N. H. Cox BSc MB ChB MRCP
Registrar in Dermatology
Western Infirmary, Glasgow
Cutaneous Infections

Andrew Y. Finlay MB BS MRCP
Senior Lecturer in Dermatology
Department of Medicine,
University of Wales College of Medicine, Cardiff;
Consultant Dermatologist, Lately:
Southern General Hospital and Western Infirmary, Glasgow
The Biology of Ageing Skin

Emily Grundy MA MSc
Lecturer in Social Gerontology
Age Concern Institute of Gerontology, King's College London (KQC),
University of London
Future Patterns of Morbidity in Old Age

J. M. Guralnik MD PhD
Research Fellow in Epidemiology
National Institute on Aging, Bethesda, USA
The Changing Demography of the Elderly in the United States

D. R. Hannay MD MRCGP
Professor of Geriatric Practice
University of Sheffield;
Lately: General Practitioner, Dumfries and Galloway
Geriatric Care in a Rural Setting

Anne P. Harrison MB ChB MRCP
Registrar in Dermatology
Royal Infirmary, Glasgow
Blistering Diseases in Old Age

R. E. Irvine OBE MD FRCP
Consultant Physician in Geriatric Medicine (retired)
Guernsey, Channel Islands
Future Developments in Geriatric Medicine

P. V. Knight MB ChB MRCP
Consultant Physician in Geriatric Medicine
Lightburn Hospital, Glasgow;
Lately: Lecturer in Geriatric Medicine, University of Glasgow
The Choice of Oral Hypoglycaemic Agent for the Elderly

W. J. MacLennan MD FRCP
Professor of Geriatric Medicine
University of Edinburgh
The Management of Hypothermia

Rona M. MacKie MD FRCP FRCPath
Professor of Dermatology
University of Glasgow
Cutaneous Malignancy in Old Age

D. T. Roberts MB ChB FRCP
Consultant Dermatologist
Western Infirmary, Glasgow
Cutaneous Infections

N. B. Simpson, MD MRCP
Consultant Dermatologist
Western Infirmary, Glasgow
Blistering Diseases in Old Age

P. J. W. Scott BSc MB ChB MRCP
Consultant Physician in Geriatric Medicine
Stobhill General Hospital, Glasgow
Adverse Reactions to Drugs in the Elderly

J. Womersley BSc MB ChB PhD DPH FFCM
Community Medicine Specialist
Greater Glasgow Health Board, Glasgow
Population Geography in an Urban Setting

M. Varghese MD
Division of Dermatology
The New York Hospital – Cornell Medical Center,
New York, USA
Modern Dressings for Leg Ulcers

Contents

Part I
DEMOGRAPHY OF THE ELDERLY

1. THE CHANGING DEMOGRAPHY OF THE ELDERLY IN THE UNITED STATES

J. M. Guralnik, D. B. Brock and J. A. Brody

In the United States in 1900 there were 3·1 million adults aged 65 and older. By 1984, that number had increased to 28 million. By all indications, this dramatic growth of the older population will continue into the next century, with substantial increases projected for both the number of persons aged 65 and older and for the number of those reaching the oldest ages.

This chapter describes current and future population characteristics, mortality, morbidity and health care utilization patterns among the elderly. These demographic changes provide a basis for understanding the enormous impact of ageing on American society.

POPULATION CHARACTERISTICS

The United States have experienced a rapid growth in the number of older people in this century. This is illustrated in *Table* 1.1, which also presents US Bureau of the Census projections through to the middle of the next century. These projections highlight two important trends: first, the impressive increase expected in the number of older persons, and second, and more important in terms of the impact that ageing will have on society, the increasing proportion of the total population who are 65 and over. Although the elderly comprised only 4 per cent of the population at the turn of the century, this figure rose to 11·3 per cent in 1980 and may be as high as 17 per cent by 2020.[1] *Table* 1.1 also illustrates that, among those aged 65 and over, the proportion of those in the 75–84 and 85 and over age-groups is increasing significantly. While those of 85 and older made up only 4 per cent of the elderly population in 1900 and 9 per cent in 1980, by the year 2040 it is projected that nearly one in five elderly persons will be over the age of 85. It can thus be seen that, in addition to the overall population getting older, the older population itself is getting older and will continue to do so.

Projections of future population size, medical problems and health care expenditure are made frequently in this chapter. It must be kept in

Table 1.1. Actual and projected growth of the older population (000s)

Year	*Total population (all ages)*	*65 years and over*		*65–74 years*		*75–84 years*		*85+ years*	
		No.	*% of all ages*	*No.*	*% of 65+*	*No.*	*% of 65+*	*No.*	*% of 65+*
1900	76,303	3,084	4·0	2,189	71·0	772	25·0	123	4·0
1920	105,711	4,933	4·7	3,464	70·2	1,259	25·5	210	4·3
1940	131,669	9,019	6·8	6,375	70·7	2,278	25·3	365	4·0
1960	179,323	16,560	9·2	10,997	66·4	4,633	28·0	929	5·6
1980	226,505	25,544	11·3	15,578	61·0	7,727	30·2	2,240	8·8
2000	267,955	34,921	13·0	17,677	50·6	12,318	35·3	4,926	14·1
2020	296,597	51,422	17·3	29,855	58·0	14,486	28·2	7,081	13·8
2040	308,559	66,988	21·7	29,272	43·7	24,882	37·1	12,834	19·2

Source: US Bureau of the Census (1984) *Decennial Censuses of Population, 1900–1980* and US Bureau of the Census (1984) Current Population Reports, Series P-25, No. 952, *Projections of the Population of the United States, by Age, Sex and Race: 1983 to 2080*. Washington, DC, US Government Printing Office.

mind that although these projections are of some interest, there is wide room for error in them. Population projections form the basis for most of the other projections and current alternative population projections vary considerably. The projections in *Table* 1.1 come from the middle series assumptions in the most recently published projections of the US Census Bureau.[1] Other mortality assumptions are also used by the Census Bureau to create alternative projections and the largest projected differences are in the size of the elderly population. The low mortality assumption made by the Census Bureau uses an estimate of annual improvement in life expectancy that is nearly twice that of the middle mortality assumption. However, even this low mortality assumption can be thought of as somewhat conservative, as it does not reflect nearly as great an annual decline in mortality rates as those that actually occurred between 1968 and 1982. Under the Census Bureau low mortality assumption, there will be 12 per cent more persons aged 65 and over in 2040 than under the middle assumption.[1] In the age group 85 and over, however, there are projected to be 17·3 million people in 2040 under the low mortality assumption compared with 12·8 million under the middle mortality assumption. Therefore, there would be 35 per cent more people than expected in this oldest age-group if mortality rates turn out to be comparable to the lower mortality assumption.

In 1920 the life expectancy of females in the USA was less than 2 years greater than that for males, but by 1984 this difference had increased to over 7 years.[2] This relative improvement in female versus male survival rates has led to an elderly population that comprises many more women than men. The dynamics of this situation can be appreciated by observing that in 1950 there were 89 men aged 65 and over for every 100 women, while by 1984 this number had dropped to 67.[3] The differences are particularly extreme at the oldest ages. In 1984 there were only 41 men for every 100 women aged 85 and older.[3] It has been projected that in the next century the ratio of elderly males to females will remain about the same for all those aged 65 and over.[4] This will result from a projected small rise in the ratio for those aged 65–84 and a moderate decline in the ratio for those aged 85 years and over. For the 85 and over age group in the coming century, there will be only 39 men for every 100 women.

There is considerable variability in the proportion of the population who are elderly among different racial and ethnic groups in the USA. The proportion of the population aged 65 and over in 1982 was about 12 per cent among whites, 8 per cent among blacks, 6 per cent among Asians and Pacific Islanders and 5 per cent among American Indians and Hispanics.[5] These figures result only partially from differential life expectancies. They are mainly affected by such factors as differential fertility rates and immigration of disproportionately higher numbers of younger people in ethnic groups characterized by a high volume of immigration. The older black population has actually grown faster than the older white population. Between 1970 and 1980 there was a 34·9 per cent increase in blacks aged 65 and over compared to a 26·7 per cent increase in whites.[6]

The geographical distribution and migration of the elderly in the USA are interesting and important issues. In 1980, the population aged 65 and over was over 2 million in both California and New York and over 1 million in Florida, Illinois, Ohio, Pennsylvania and Texas.[6] These seven states contained 45 per cent of all persons in this age-group. Between 1970 and 1980 there was a 27·9 per cent increase in older Americans, but this increase varied widely by geographical region. The South had a 41·1 per cent increase, the West a 39·1 per cent increase and the Northeastern and North Central states had increases of 17·3 per cent. Nevada's elderly population increased during this time by 114 per cent, Arizona's by 91 per cent, Hawaii's by 73 per cent and Florida's by 71 per cent. These figures represent a migration from the Northeast and Central states to the West and South, but it is important to note that the overall rate of interstate migration for those 65 and over is relatively low. Between 1975 and 1979, 3·6 per cent of older people moved from one state to another while 8·1 per cent of the population aged 4 years and over made a move of this type.

Family composition and living arrangements among those aged 65 years and over are influenced most strongly by the differential mortality experienced by men and women. *Fig.* 1.1 shows rates of widowhood by age, race and sex in 1982. For those aged 75 and over, black females have the highest rate, with nearly 80 per cent widowed, while white males have the lowest rate, with only 20·6 per cent widowed. Overall, the most common living arrangement for elderly persons is to live with their spouse in a household with no other persons, but this situation varies greatly by sex and age. In 1980, 74 per cent of older men but only 36 per cent of older women had a spouse present in the household.[6] For those aged 75 and over, 65 per cent of men compared with 19 per cent of women had a spouse present in the household. As stated earlier, in the next century the male/female ratio for those aged 85 and over is expected to continue to decline. As a result, the proportion of these oldest women who live with a spouse will become extremely small.

Family support may play an important role in aiding the older person with such things as maintaining a healthy lifestyle, complying with medical treatment and avoiding admission to a nursing home. One method of estimating the availability of family support for older persons is to examine the ratio of those in older age-groups in comparison with middle age-groups. As the postwar baby boom generation reaches middle age at the turn of the century, this ratio will

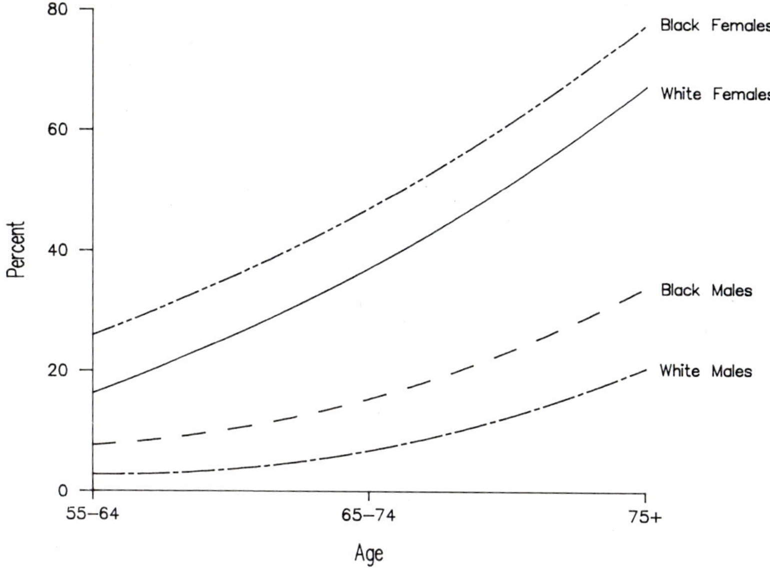

Fig. 1.1. Widowhood of persons aged 55 and over by race and sex, United States, 1982.
Source: US Bureau of the Census (1983) Current Population Reports, Series P-20, No. 380, *Marital Status and Living Arrangements: March 1982*. Washington, DC, US Government Printing Office.

drop, with more support available for those aged 65 and over. By the third decade of the next century, however, this situation will change significantly. At that time, the combination of the baby boom generation passing age 65 and the lower fertility rates seen in the 1960s and 1970s will cause a substantial rise in this ratio.[6] A situation may thus be anticipated where less social and economic support, especially for women, will come from spouses or children, but will instead be required from the community.

In the past 20 years, striking increases have occurred in the numbers and sizes of nursing homes, with the creation of a large nursing home industry in the USA. The utilization of nursing homes has been affected by many of the previously discussed demographic trends, such as changes in survival and family composition, as well as by the availability of public financing under the Medicaid programme, begun in the mid-1960s. In 1963, half a million elderly people representing 2·5 per cent of the older US population, resided in nursing homes. By 1981 this number had tripled to 1·4 million people, or 5·3 per cent of those aged 65 and above.[6] The institutionalization rates for older women and men were respectively 6·3 and 3·8 per cent.

THE OLDEST OLD

In observing the phenomenon of the ageing population, it is of particular interest to look at those aged 85 and over, recently termed 'the oldest old'.[7] This group constitutes the most rapidly growing segment of the American population. While the total US population increased by 26 per cent between 1960 and 1980, those aged 85 and over increased by 126 per cent.[8] In actual numbers, the oldest old are expected to increase from 2·2 million in 1980 to 4·9 million by 2000 and 7·1 million by 2020.[1]

Rapid changes in the older population are most acutely apparent when observing changes in the oldest old population. In just 4 years, between 1980 and 1984, the total population aged 85 and over increased from 2·24 million to 2·67 million, an astounding 19 per cent increase.[3] With changes as profound as this, it is clear that understanding the current situation and accurately projecting the future will depend in great measure on the frequent updating of demographic, health and health care utilization data on the population of older persons.

A substantially increased burden of poor health in the oldest old, as compared to all people aged 65 and over, is demonstrated by a variety of health status indicators, including measures of chronic diseases, disabilities and use of medical services. Male/female differences in survival, widowhood, living arrangements and institutionalization are even more pronounced in this group than in the 65 and over age-group in general. The oldest old represent the segment of our population with the highest per capita needs for medical services and nursing home care, and the future growth that has been projected for this group will undoubtedly have a marked impact on the health care delivery system.

MORTALITY AND SURVIVAL

Dramatic changes in mortality occurring in this century have led to increased life expectancy at all ages, although the gains for older persons have come mainly in the past 40 years (*Table* 1.2). Between 1900 and 1940, overall life expectancy increased by nearly 14 years while life expectancy for those aged 65 increased by less than 1 year. Mortality rates for older persons dropped between 1940 and 1954, rose slightly between 1954 and 1968 and then fell again from 1968 through to 1982.[9] This is seen in the gains in life expectancy of nearly 2 years between 1940 and 1954 and of over 2 years between 1968 and 1983 for those aged 65 years.

The gains seen in life expectancy during this century have not been uniform for males and females and for whites and blacks. *Table* 1.2

illustrates how the male/female difference in survival has increased during this century. A 65-year-old white female could expect to live only 0·7 years longer than a 65-year-old white male at the turn of the century, 1·5 years longer in 1940, but over 4 years longer in 1983. While life expectancy at birth has consistently been higher for whites than for blacks, this advantage is not seen for those reaching age 65 or over. In fact an 80-year-old black person has a slightly longer remaining life expectancy than a white person of similar age.

Table 1.2. Average remaining lifetime at various ages, by sex and race, 1900–1983

	1983	*1968*	*1954*	*1939–1941*	*1929–1931*	*1900–1902*
All classes						
At birth	74·6	70·2	69·6	63·6	59·3	49·2
65 years	16·7	14·6	14·4	12·6	12·3	11·9
75 years	10·7	9·1	9·0	7·6	7·3	7·1
80 years	8·1	6·8	6·9	5·7	5·4	5·3
Whites						
Male						
At birth	71·7	67·5	67·4	62·8	59·1	48·2
65 years	14·5	12·8	13·1	12·1	11·8	11·5
75 years	9·0	8·1	8·2	7·2	7·0	6·8
80 years	6·9	6·2	6·3	5·4	5·3	5·1
Female						
At birth	78·7	74·9	73·6	67·3	62·7	51·1
65 years	18·7	16·4	15·7	13·6	12·8	12·2
75 years	11·8	9·8	9·4	7·9	7·6	7·3
80 years	8·8	7·0	7·0	5·9	5·6	5·5
Blacks and other races*						
Male						
At birth	67·2	60·1	61·0	52·3	47·6	32·5
65 years	14·1	12·1	13·5	12·2	10·9	10·4
75 years	9·4	9·9	10·4	8·2	7·0	6·6
80 years	7·4	8·7	9·1	6·6	5·4	5·1
Female						
At birth	74·9	67·5	65·8	55·6	49·5	35·0
65 years	17·9	15·1	15·7	13·9	12·2	11·4
75 years	11·9	11·5	12·0	9·8	8·6	7·9
80 years	9·3	9·3	10·1	8·0	6·9	6·5

* Blacks only for 1900–1902 and 1929–1931.

Source: US Bureau of the Census (1984) Current Population Reports, Series P-23, No. 138, *Demographic and Socioeconomic Aspects of Aging in the United States*. Washington, DC, US Government Printing Office. National Center for Health Statistics (1985) *Advance Report of Final Mortality Statistics, 1983*. *Monthly Vital Statistics Report*, Vol. 34, No. 6. Suppl. (2). DHHS Pub. No. (PHS) 85-120. Hyattsville, Md, Public Health Service.

Diseases of the heart are by far the most frequently occurring cause of death for those aged 65 and over, leading to 44 per cent of all deaths and causing more than twice as many deaths as the second leading cause of death, malignant neoplasms.[10] Cerebrovascular disease is the third leading cause of death in older persons, followed bypneumonia, influenza and arteriosclerosis. Cardiovascular diseases thus make up three of the five leading causes of death for older persons. The importance of cardiovascular diseases in ageing is clearly illustrated in *Fig.* 1.2. Cardiovascular disease mortality rises steeply with increasing age and resembles the all-cause mortality curve. This is quite different from the curve representing death rates from all cancers, which rises quite modestly in older ages.

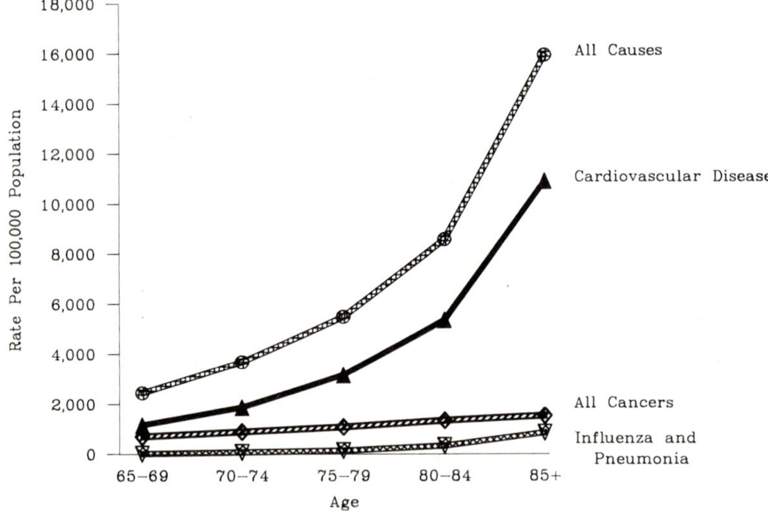

Fig. 1.2. Mortality rates per 100 000 for selected causes, United States, 1980. *Source*: National Center for Health Statistics (1985) *Vital Statistics of the United States, 1980, Vol. II, Mortality, Part A*. DHHS Pub. No. (PHS) 85-1101. Public Health Service. Washington, DC, US Government Printing Office.

The decline in mortality seen in older persons in the past 40 years has in large part been due to a decline in cardiovascular diseases. The decline in mortality from heart disease accounted for half of the decline in overall mortality rates between 1950 and 1979, while the decline in stroke mortality accounted for one-quarter of the overall decline.[10] Cancer was the only major cause of death to increase during this period.

Recent declines in mortality in the US elderly have been more rapid than for older persons in all other countries except Japan.[10] Future declines in mortality will depend on a continued drop in heart disease and stroke, the driving forces in recent declines, or a turnaround and subsequent decline in death rates for cancer, the second leading cause of death. A theoretical means of evaluating the impact of a specific disease on mortality is to evaluate the gain in life expectancy that might be realized if that disease were eliminated as a cause of death. The elimination of all cardiovascular diseases would result in a 14·3-year gain in life expectancy for those aged 65 and over, while the elimination of heart disease alone would lead to a gain of 6·6 years.[6] The elimination of malignant neoplasms as a group would lead to a 3·1-year gain in life expectancy from birth but, since this cause affects such a wide range of ages, only a 1·9-year gain for those who have survived to age 65. Hence, the potential gain in life expectancy for older persons from the elimination of malignant neoplasms is substantially less than for cardiovascular disease.

Morbidity

Several different types of measures can be useful in representing the health status of the elderly: (1) health care utilization patterns such as hospital days and physician visits, (2) incidence and prevalence rates of

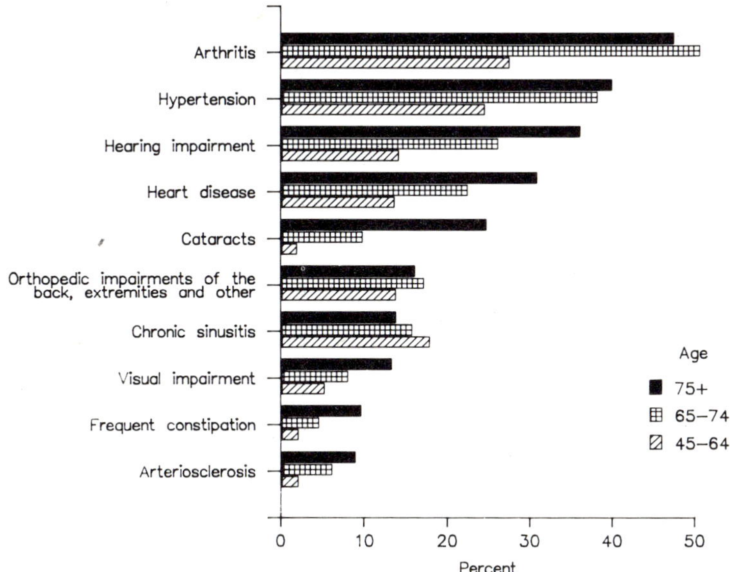

Fig. 1.3. Prevalence of leading chronic conditions, United States, 1982. *Source*: National Center for Health Statistics (1985) *Current estimates from the National Health Interview Survey, United States, 1982*. DHHS Pub. No. (PHS) 85-1578. Public Health Service. Washington, DC, US Government Printing Office.

specific diseases and conditions, and (3) indicators of functional status or disability. This section focuses on disease and disability measures; health care utilization is discussed later.

Prevalence rates are shown in *Fig.* 1.3 for diseases and health conditions most frequently reported by those aged 45–64, 65–74 and 75 and over. This figure demonstrates a substantial amount of prevalent morbidity in older persons. Arthritis is reported by nearly half of those aged 65 and over and is nearly twice as prevalent as among those aged 45–64. Hypertension is reported by over one-third of those aged 65 and over, while over one-quarter have hearing impairments and heart conditions. For many of these conditions the prevalence rises substantially with age. For other conditions (arthritis, hypertension, orthopaedic impairments and chronic sinusitis), the rates are no higher in those aged 75 and over when compared with the 65–74-year-old age-group.

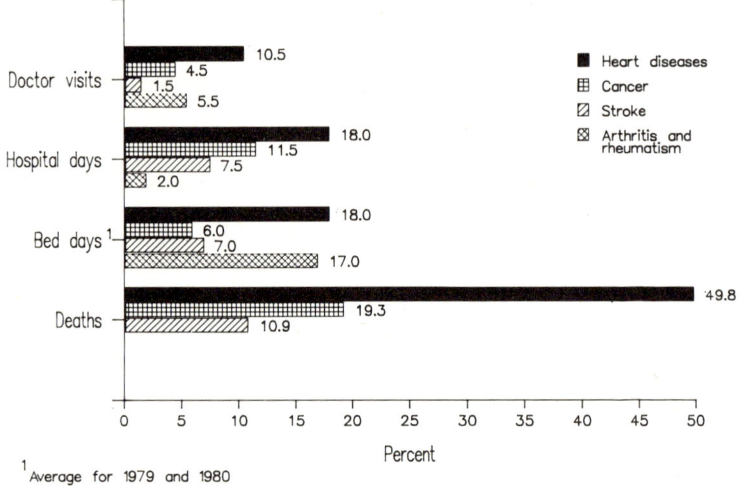

Fig. 1.4. Burden of illness resulting from selected conditions in persons 65 years of age and older, United States, 1980.
Source: National Center for Health Statistics (1982) *Health, United States, 1982*. DHHS Pub. No. (PHS) 83-1232. Public Health Service. Washington, DC, US Government Printing Office, and National Center for Health Statistics (1985) *Vital Statistics of the United States, 1980, Vol. II, Mortality, Part A*. DHHS Pub. No. (PHS) 85-1101. Public Health Service. Washington, DC, US Government Printing Office.

The burden of illness resulting from important conditions affecting the elderly is illustrated in *Fig.* 1.4. Heart disease is responsible for more doctor visits, hospital days, bed days and deaths than the other major causes of morbidity in the elderly, namely cancer, stroke and

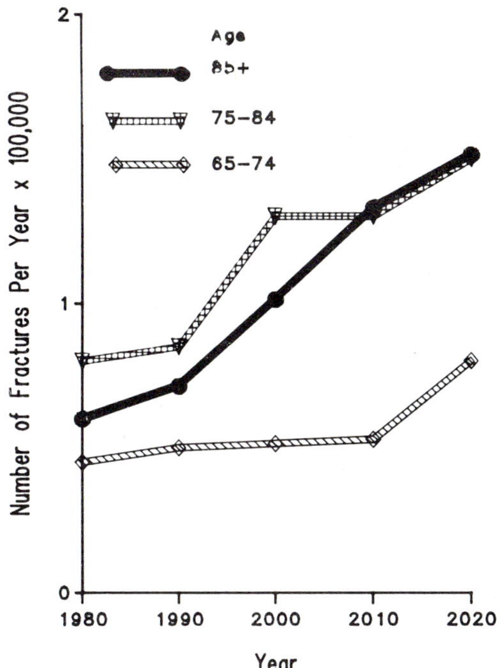

Fig. 1.5. Projected number of hip fractures annually in the United States by age, 1980–2020.
Source: Farmer M. E., White L. R., Brody J. A. et al. (1984) *Am. J. Public Health* **74**, 1374, and US Bureau of the Census (1982) Current Population Reports, Series P-25, No. 922, *Projections of the Population of the United States: 1982 to 2050* (Advance Report). Washington, DC, US Government Printing Office.

arthritis. Arthritis and rheumatism in the elderly account for more bed days than cancer and stroke and nearly as many bed days as heart disease.

As difficult as is the prediction of future mortality rates, the prediction of future morbidity is much more problematic. Shifts in the age structure of the elderly population, changes in health habits and health care and scientific breakthroughs will all have a significant impact on future morbidity levels. The simple growth of the older population will lead to substantially more cases of all diseases that affect the elderly. *Figs.* 1.5 and 1.6 show the projected number of cases in the USA for two important conditions affecting the elderly—hip fracture and dementia. These projections use the assumption that age-specific incidence rates for these conditions will remain the same in the future. The rapid rise in the number of cases in those aged 85 and over reflects a combination of both the high incidence rates and the rapid growth in this age-group.

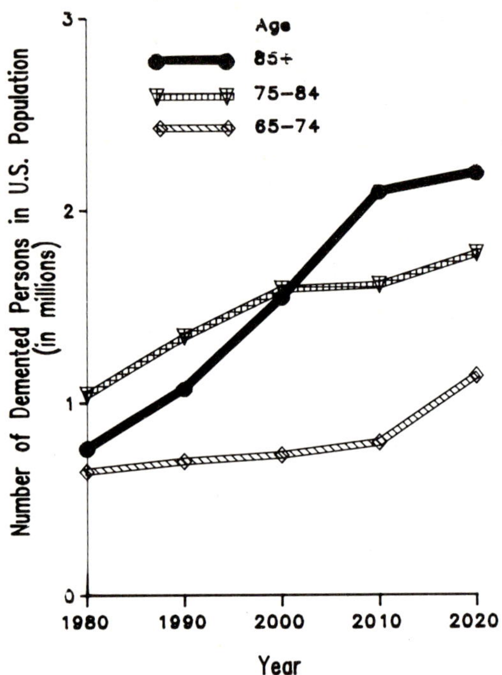

Fig. 1.6. Projected number of demented persons in the United States by age, 1980–2020.
Source: National Institute on Aging, Prevalence Estimates, and US Bureau of the Census (1982) Current Population Reports, Series P-25, No. 922, *Projections of the Population of the United States: 1982 to 2050* (Advance Report). Washington, DC, US Government Printing Office.

With the high prevalence of chronic conditions and the frequent occurrence of multiple conditions in older persons, a valuable indicator of morbidity may be obtained by using measures of functional status to characterize the overall impact of one or more diseases or conditions on the individual. The evaluation of activities of daily living (ADL) is commonly used to identify serious declines in physical functioning. *Table* 1.3 shows the percentage of those needing help, by age and sex, in one or more of the following activities: walking, bathing, dressing, eating, getting into and out of bed, and using the toilet. Of note in these data are the steep increase in disability with age and the increased levels of disability in women compared to men in each age-group of 65 and over.

An important question in the study of ageing is whether gains in health status accompany the gains in life expectancy that are now occurring and are expected to continue. The implications of this question are momentous. The impact on the health care system and society in general will be very different if added years of life result from an extension of life in those already seriously ill as opposed to the added years resulting from a postponement of severe, debilitating diseases.

Table 1.3. Morbidity measures by age and sex

Age and sex	*Percentage with limitations in ADL**	*Rates per 1000 per year* Hospital days of care	*Physician visits*	*Percentage in nursing homes*
Male				
Total	1·3	1053·4	4048·0	0·36
Under 20	0·2	357·0	4224·3	
20–44	0·4	608·4	3231·0	0·09
45–64	1·9	1587·9	4388·0	
65+	6·8	4243·9	5925·8	3·07
65–74	4·4	3370·0	5539·5	1·27
75–84	9·7	5476·4	6799·3	4·74
85 and over	21·7	7674·4	6362·0	14·00
Female				
Total	1·9	1355·0	5413·0	0·84
Under 20	0·2	388·7	4294·2	
20–44	0·5	1070·0	5739·1	0·10
45–64	1·8	1604·0	5679·7	
65+	10·4	3999·8	6763·5	5·97
65–74	5·1	2977·3	7018·7	1·59
75–84	15·0	5009·0	6524·8	8·06
85 and over	34·6	6598·9	5677·8	25·15

* Limitations in one or more activities of daily living (ADL): walking, bathing, dressing, eating, getting in and out of bed and using the toilet.
Source: National Center for Health Statistics, in Rice D. P. and Feldman J. J. (1983) *Milbank Mem. Fund Q.* **61**, 362.

In attempting to answer this question it is necessary to evaluate changes in morbidity in the older population over time. There are particular problems in using more conventional measures of morbidity, such as disease incidence or health care utilization, to assess long-term changes in morbidity. Changes in reporting of disease may be strongly influenced by increased access to medical care or changes in medical practice in the community. Trends in hospitalizations or admissions to nursing homes may be a result of changes in health care financing policies. Measuring functional status, in which an individual's ability to perform specific tasks is evaluated, probably offers the best way to evaluate morbidity change. A potentially important tool that uses this approach is the calculation of expected remaining years of disability-free life, also termed 'active life expectancy'. Using a longitudinal study of older persons in Massachusetts, Katz and colleagues computed active life expectancy, which they defined as the expected number of years of remaining life in which one remains independent (needs no help) in performing ADL.[11] Women, as expected, were shown to have a longer life expectancy at all ages, but in terms of active life expectancy, women showed only a modest advantage over men in the 65–69 age-group and no advantage in the older groups. The important finding in this research is that although women consistently live longer than men, the number of years that elderly women spend disabled is greater and the total non-disabled life expectancy for men and women who have reached age 65 is similar. An analysis using population statistics for Canada showed similar results.[12] Using data collected in 1950–1951 for comparison, this study was also able to demonstrate that only part of the increase in life expectancy that has occurred in the past 30 years has been accompanied by an increase in disability-free life. Between 1950–1951 and 1978, life expectancy rose 4·5 years for males and 7·5 years for females, while expected years of disability-free life rose by only 1·3 and 1·4 years respectively.

HEALTH CARE UTILIZATION

With the increase in the number and proportion of elderly persons in our society, it is important to consider projected increases in health care utilization. Recent rates for the USA for the three main areas of utilization—physician care, hospital care and nursing home care—are shown in *Table* 1.3. Hospital utilization rises steadily with age, but physician visits are fewer among those aged 85 and over compared with the next younger group. Overall, about 5 per cent of those aged 65 and over reside in nursing homes at any one time. However, there are substantial sex differences found for institutionalization, with rates being respectively 3·1 and 6·0 per cent for elderly men and women. Particularly striking is the fact that 14 per cent of men and 25 per cent of women aged 85 and over are confined to nursing homes. It has been clearly demonstrated that the lifetime risk of institutionalization is much higher than the point prevalence of nursing home residency, but there has been debate over just how high this risk is. Estimates of the probability of a 65-year-old in the USA being institutionalized in a nursing home at some time prior to death range from 24 to 48 per cent.[13,14,15,16]

The proportion of health care resources used by older persons is a reflection of their poorer health status. The elderly comprised 11 per cent of the US population in 1981, but 33 per cent of the health care dollar was spent for their care. Compared to the $828 spent yearly on health care by persons under age 65, persons aged 65 and over spent $3140 per capita, or more than three and a half times as much.[17]

Projections of the future utilization of health care services and the cost of these services constitute a complex process, dependent on many variables. Projections of more than just a few years into the future are full of uncertainties and must be viewed with caution. Making the assumption that age-specific rates of health care utilization would remain stable, Rice and Feldman projected future physician visits, hospital and nursing home care and health care expenditure.[18] Rates of physician visits do not vary as much by age as do those of hospital or nursing home utilization. Consequently, the increase in physician visits due to ageing of the population will be considerably smaller than increases in other measures of utilization. Between 1980 and 2020, the total number of short-stay hospital days is projected to rise from 274 million to 459 million days. More than 65 per cent of this increase is projected to be due to hospitalization in the expanding population of older persons. In 2020 it is projected that 28 per cent of days of care will be for those aged 75 and above compared with 20 per cent in 1980. Assuming that older persons need greater intensity of care, these figures imply that there will be significant increases not only in the number of hospital days but in the expenditure per day.

As might be expected, the ageing of the population has a much greater impact on nursing home utilization than on hospital care days or physician visits. *Fig.* 1.7 illustrates the projected number of elderly persons in nursing homes through to the year 2020. The total number of older persons in nursing homes is projected to rise from 1·3 million in 1980 to about 2·9 million in 2020. The increase in numbers is again seen to be most dramatic for those aged 85 and over, with an expected rise from 0·5 million nursing home residents in 1980 to 1·6 million in 2020. The oldest old age-group now comprises less than 40 per cent of the elderly nursing home population. By 2020, due to the rapid growth and high rate of nursing home utilization of the oldest old population, 55 per cent of all elderly people in nursing homes will be aged 85 and over.

Reflecting the utilization of medical services, the proportional increase in medical expenditure is expected to rise far more sharply among older persons. *Table* 1.4 illustrates the projected increases in total health care expenditure and nursing home expenditure between 1980 and 2020. In constant 1980 dollars, total expenditure is expected to rise 100 per cent for those aged 65 and over but only 18 per cent for all those under 65.

These figures offer a sobering view of the impact of the ageing population on the health care system. Projections presented here were generated on the assumption that health status within each age-group of the elderly will remain constant in the future. One hope for a more

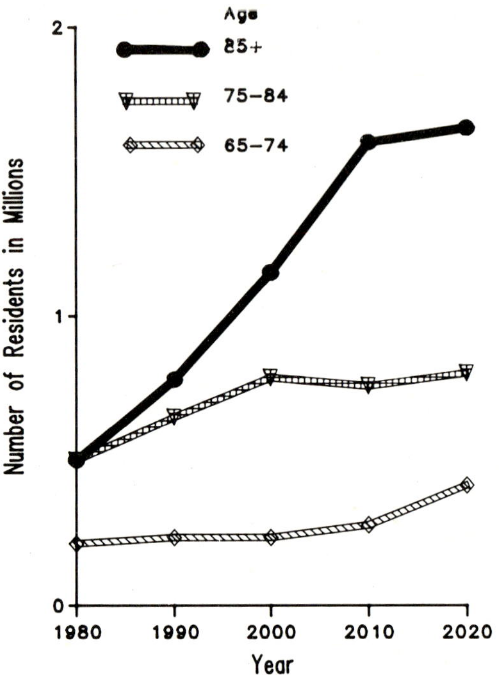

Fig. 1.7. Projected number of nursing home residents in the United States by age, 1980–2020.
Source: National Center for Health Statistics (1979) *The National Nursing Home Survey*, 1977 summary for the United States. DHEW Pub. No. (PHS) 79-1794. Public Health Service. Washington, DC, US Government Printing Office, and US Bureau of the Census (1982) Current Population Reports, Series P-25, No. 922, *Projections of the Population of the United States: 1982 to 2050* (Advance Report), Washington, DC, US Government Printing Office.

Table 1.4. Projected personal health care and nursing home expenditure by age, United States, 1980–2020*

Age	*1980*	*2000*	*2020*
Total expenditure			
All ages	$219·4	$273·4	$328·3
Under 19 years of age	25·9	26·9	28·1
19–64 years of age	129·0	156·2	169·0
65 years and over	64·5	90·3	131·2
Nursing home expenditure			
All ages	$ 20·6	$ 28·0	$ 38·9
Under 19 years of age	0·1	0·1	0·1
19–64 years of age	4·0	4·8	5·2
65 years and over	16·5	23·1	33·6

* Figures denote billions, in constant 1980 dollars.
Source: Rice D. P. and Feldman J. J. (1983) *Milbank Mem. Fund Q.* **61**, 362.

favourable picture to emerge is that better health practices in the population which is now young, along with advances in disease prevention and treatment, will lead to a generally healthier older population in the future.

CONCLUSION

Since the beginning of this century, the elderly population in the United States has experienced an eightfold increase in absolute numbers, and the overall proportion of elderly persons has tripled. A person reaching the age of 65 today can expect to live for 16 more years, and numerous factors affect the quality of life during those years. The increased survival of women compared to men results in far larger numbers of women who are widowed and living alone or institutionalized. The high prevalence of chronic diseases and the frequent coexistence of multiple conditions result in rising rates of disability as people age. Those aged 85 and above, a rapidly expanding group, are affected by particularly high rates of chronic disease, disability, hospitalization and institutionalization.

By all indications there will be a continued and rapid growth of the elderly population well into the twenty-first century. As demonstrated in this chapter, the impact of this growth will result from two important factors. First, the absolute size of the elderly population will nearly triple by 2040 and will, more importantly, make up a substantially larger proportion of the total population, changing from 11 to 22 per cent. Second, the age structure of the elderly population itself will shift significantly and will comprise higher proportions of very old persons. In the face of these important demographic changes, there are clear and compelling challenges to geriatric medicine and society as a whole to prevent or postpone disease and disability and to care more effectively for older persons.

REFERENCES

1. US Bureau of the Census (1984) *Projections of the Population of the United States by Age, Sex and Race: 1983 to 2080*. Current Population Reports, Series P-25, No. 952. Washington, DC, US Government Printing Office.
2. National Center for Health Statistics (1986) *Advance Report of Final Mortality Statistics, 1984. Monthly Vital Statistics Report*, Vol. 35, No. 6, Suppl. (2). DHHS Publication No. (PHS) 86-1120. Hyattsville, Md, Public Health Service.
3. US Bureau of the Census (1985) *Estimates of the Population of the United States by Age, Sex and Race: 1980 to 1984*. Current Population Reports, Series P-25, No. 965. Washington, DC, US Government Printing Office.
4. Seigel J. S. (1980) In: Haynes S. G. and Feinleib M. (eds) *Second Conference on the Epidemiology of Aging*. NIH Publication No. 80-969. Washington, DC, US Government Printing Office.

5. US Bureau of the Census (1983) America in Transition: An Aging Society. Current Population Reports, Series P-23, No. 128. Washington, DC, US Government Printing Office.
6. US Bureau of the Census (1984) *Demographic and Socioeconomic Aspects of Aging in the United States*, Current Population Reports, Series P-23, No. 138. Washington, DC, US Government Printing Office.
7. Suzman R. and Riley M. W. (1985) *Milbank Mem. Fund Q.* **63**, 177.
8. Rosenswaike I. (1985) *Milbank Mem. Fund Q.* **63**, 187.
9. Social Security Administration, Office of the Actuary (1985) *Social Security Area Population Projections, 1985*. Actuarial Study No. 95, SSA Publication No. 11-11542.
10. National Center for Health Statistics (1982) *Health, United States, 1982*. DHHS Publication No. (PHS) 83-1232, Public Health Service. Washington, DC, US Government Printing Office.
11. Katz S., Branch L. G., Branson M. H. et al. (1983) *N. Engl. J. Med.* **309**, 1218.
12. Wilkins R. and Adams O. B. (1983) *Am. J. Public Health.* **73**, 1073.
13. Kastenbaum R. S. and Candy S. (1977) *Int. J. Aging Hum. Dev.* **4**, 303.
14. McConnel C. E. (1984) *Gerontologist* **24**, 193.
15. Palmore E. (1976) *Gerontologist* **16**, 504.
16. Vicente L., Wiley J. and Carrington R. A. (1979) *Gerontologist* **19**, 52.
17. US Senate Special Committee on Aging (1985) *Aging America, Trends and Projections*. Washington, DC, US Government Printing Office.
18. Rice D. R. and Feldman J. J. (1983) Milbank Mem. Fund Q. **61**, 362.

2. POPULATION GEOGRAPHY IN AN URBAN SETTING

J. Womersley

INTRODUCTION

The aim of this chapter is to describe the characteristics of all the people aged 65 years and over who live within the area served by a large, mainly urban, health authority, and to provide some indication of their needs and the extent to which these are met—or, often, fail to be met—by health services. Emphasis is given to demonstrating geographical variability within the authority, and to stressing the desirability of taking these differences into account when planning services.

DESCRIPTION OF THE GREATER GLASGOW HEALTH BOARD AREA

The area served by the Greater Glasgow Health Board (GGHB) extends to some 55 000 hectares (132 000 acres) and has a population of just under 1 million (986 818) or about one-fifth of the population of Scotland. It comprises five local government districts, about three-quarters of its population living in Glasgow City (755 429) with the remainder living in Clydebank, Bearsden and Milngavie, Strathkelvin and Eastwood. Although the area is predominantly urban, there are substantial rural components outside Glasgow City.

The present urban centre was laid out near the north bank of the Clyde as a residential neighbourhood to the west of the original mediaeval township of Glasgow; this was at a time of prosperous mercantile development during the eighteenth century. The city grew concentrically from its origins, incorporating previously outlying settlements, particularly during the rapid expansion of mainly heavy industry in the nineteenth century. The new housing was predominantly tenemental, and there was severe overcrowding of housing in the central areas.

In the following century, the interwar housing schemes were the first large-scale attempts by local government to meet the chronic housing needs of the city. They were developed largely on peripheral green-field areas, and included the well-planned schemes of Knightswood, Riddrie and Mosspark and the later and less attractive schemes such as Blackhill.

During the postwar period more peripheral schemes were built, for example Drumchapel, Nitshill, Pollok, Castlemilk, Ruchazie, Garthamlock and Easterhouse. A common failing in these areas was the lack of community amenities, some of which were not built for many years. Although this problem has been alleviated, these schemes are generally unattracive and suffer from a combination of bad planning, housing in poor repair or vacant, poor amenity provision, high transport costs and social problems such as low incomes and high unemployment.

The other main features of postwar housing development were the extensive demolition and redevelopment of inner-city areas with high-density and relatively poor-quality tenements. This started in the Hutchesontown–Gorbals area in 1957. New, usually multi-storey, housing replaced much of the older tenemental property and more recently many of the remaining gap sites have been taken over by private housing development. Since the late 1970s considerable refurbishment has taken place of old tenemental and newer council housing.

The high level of provision of council housing in Glasgow City meant that much twentieth-century owner-occupied housing development took place beyond the city limits. Such suburban developments, of different ages, are characteristic of Bearsden, Milngavie and Bishopbriggs to the north and Cathcart, Giffnock and Clarkston to the south. Suburban areas have also developed around separate urban communities such as Kirkintilloch, Lenzie and Newton Mearns.

The area served by the greater Glasgow Health Board thus includes inner-city, rural and suburban populations of very different types. The range of social conditions includes both the most deprived and the most affluent areas, and represents in microcosm almost the full spectrum of social circumstances found in the United Kingdom.

SPATIAL DISTRIBUTION OF THE ELDERLY POPULATION

Figs. 2.1 and 2.2 show the spatial distribution of the elderly people, in this instance defined as those aged 75 years and over, who are resident in private households within the GGHB area. The small-scale map (*Fig*. 2.1) shows the entire GGHB area; 77 per cent of the GGHB population live in Glasgow City, and *Fig*. 2.2 is a larger-scale map of this particular district. The small areas on the map are postcode sectors (e.g. G12(8)), of which there are 138 entirely or mainly within the GGHB area. For the purpose of constructing these maps the postcode sectors have been ranked from lowest to highest for the criteria under consideration, and subdivided accordingly into five groups or 'quintiles' of 27 or 28 postcode sectors. *Figs*. 2.1 and 2.2 show that the

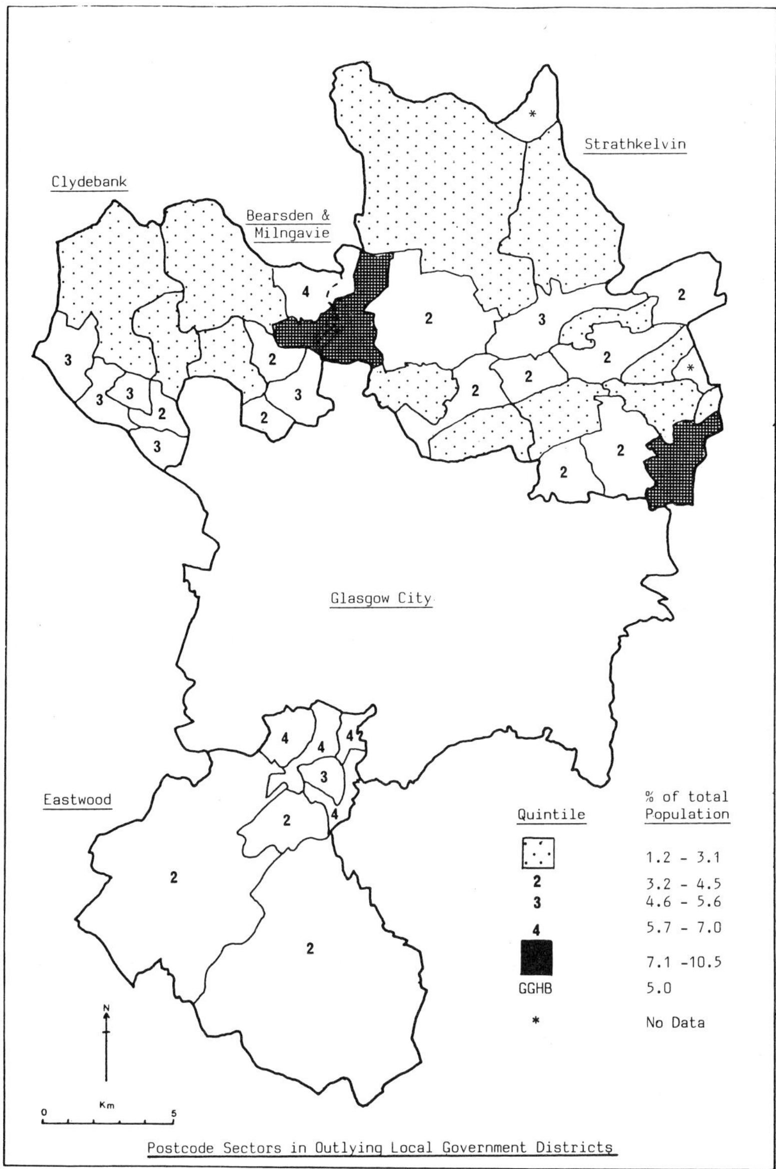

Fig. 2.1. Distribution of the elderly population (aged 75 and over) in private households within the GGHB area.

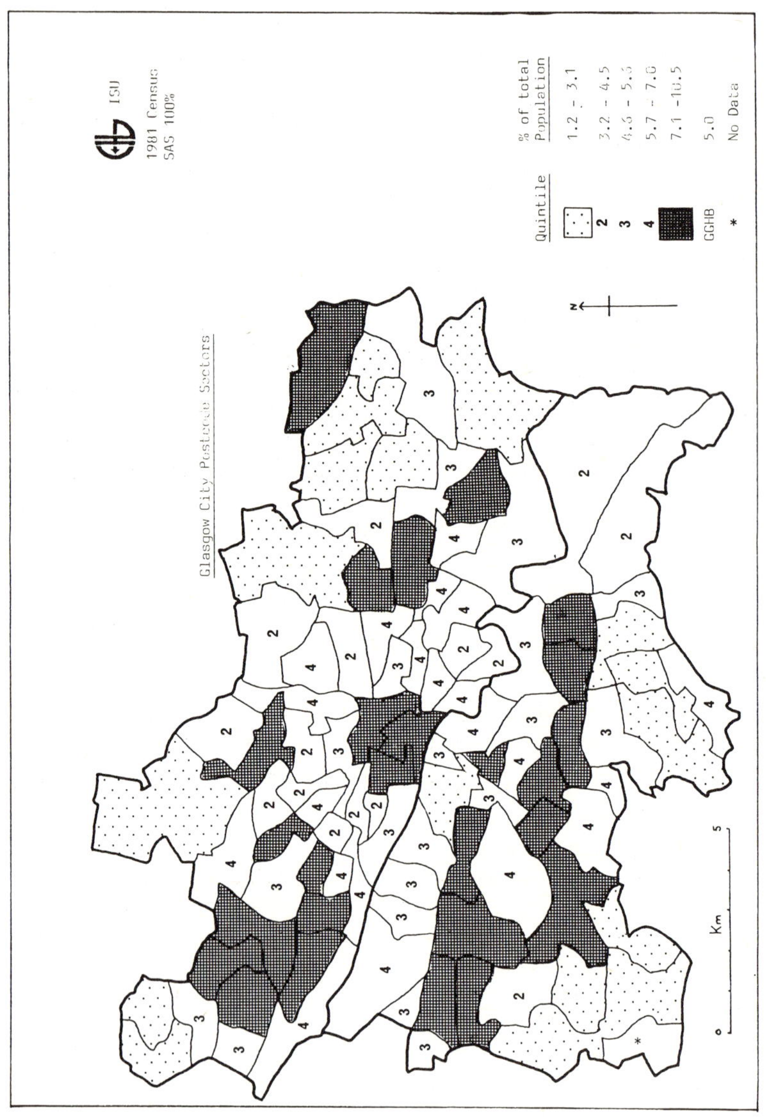

Fig. 2.2. Distribution of the elderly population (aged 75 and over) in private households in Glasgow City.

percentage of elderly people as a proportion of the population resident in the 28 postcode sectors in the lowest quintile (marked with dots) is in the range 1·2–3·1 per cent, whereas for the highest quintile (dark hatched) the range is 7·1–10·5 per cent, or about four times greater. The concentration of elderly in the population is greatest in Glasgow City (there are only two postcode sectors in the other four districts in the highest quintile). Comparison with other maps (not shown) indicates that the elderly predominate in areas of older housing—particularly in areas of relatively good-quality local authority housing in neighbourhoods towards the periphery of the city, but also in the few areas of owner-occupied housing within the city, and in areas close to the city centre where there is a relatively high proportion of privately rented accomodation. The circumstances of the elderly population are thus extremely variable. In some areas of the city over 20 per cent of people over the age of 75 years live in privately rented accommodation; in others less than 1 per cent do so. Similarly there are areas of the city where over 80 per cent of the elderly live in houses which are 'underoccupied' (having more room than a theoretical minimum requirement), whereas in other areas 10 per cent of the elderly population are living in extremely overcrowded conditions.

PRIVATE HOUSEHOLDS AND COMMUNAL ESTABLISHMENTS

Table 2.1 is an analysis according to age-group of numbers of people aged 65 years and over who at the time of the 1981 Census were normally resident in private households or in institutions in the GGHB area.

Table 2.1. Analysis by place of usual residence

Age-group (years)	*Total*	*Institutions*		*Own home*	
		No.	*% of total*	*No.*	*% living alone*
65–75	91 460	2180	2·4	89 280	30
75–84	44 716	2885	6·5	41 831	46
85+	8 783	1791	20·4	6992	42
Total	144 959	6856	4·7	138 103	

The population of the GGHB area was 986 818 and of these 145 000 (14·7 per cent) were aged 65 years and over: 63 per cent were aged 65–74 years, 31 per cent 75–84 years and 6 per cent were aged 85 years and over. The proportions normally resident in institutions for these three age-groups were respectively 2·4, 6·5 and 20·4 per cent.

Of those who lived in their own home the proportions who lived alone were respectively 30, 46 and 42 per cent for the three age-groups. Of the 6856 aged 65 years and over who were normally resident in communal establishments 54 per cent lived in long-stay hospitals (29 per cent psychiatric, 22 per cent geriatric and 3 per cent non-NHS), 34 per cent in old persons' homes, 7 per cent in hostels and common lodging homes, 3 per cent in hotels and boarding houses and 2 per cent elsewhere.

USE OF RESOURCES BY THE ELDERLY

Acute Hospital Beds

At any one time in the GGHB area there are about 1600 patients aged 65 and over occupying acute hospital beds: about 400 between the ages of 65 and 69 years, 800 between the ages of 70 and 79 years, 400 between the ages of 80 and 89 years, and 60 aged 90 years and over.

Between 1961 and 1978 the proportion of discharges from acute hospital wards (i.e. non-maternity, non-mental, non-geriatric beds) that related to patients aged 65 years and over rose from 16 to 26 per cent. However, the average length of stay for older patients is much longer than for those under 65 years: 21 days (in 1978) for those aged 75 years and over, and 14 days for those aged between 65 and 74 years, compared with 8 days for younger patients. Thus the proportion of bed days attributed to the elderly increased from 31 per cent in 1969 to 44 per cent in 1978 (20·5 per cent for the age-group 65–74 years, and 23·3 per cent for those aged 75 years and over), and to almost 50 per cent in 1984.

There is, however, considerable variation between specialties, with the elderly people (aged 65 years and over) in 1984 accounting for 55 per cent of the use of beds in the specialty of general medicine, 52 per cent of orthopaedic beds, 43 per cent of general surgery beds but only 14 per cent of gynaecology beds. The proportion of operations carried out in elderly patients has also increased: from about 14 per cent in 1968 to 17 per cent in 1974 and to 23 per cent in 1982. The increasing use of beds by the elderly is at least in part due to an increase in the number of very old people in the population, and to a general reduction in the length of stay that is most marked in the younger age-groups.

Analysis, by area of residence, of admission to acute hospitals shows an approximately twofold variation in admission rates of the elderly between those 28 postcode sectors with the highest and those 28 with the lowest admission rates. The areas with the highest admission rates lie exclusively in the most deprived inner-city areas and in one particular peripheral housing scheme, whereas the areas with the lowest admission rates are the most affluent parts of the city and suburbs.

Beds in Psychogeriatric Hospitals

According to the 1981 Census just over 2000 GGHB residents aged 65 years and over are normally resident in long-term psychiatric hospitals (including about 170 people in hospitals for the mentally handicapped). About 63 per cent of these individuals are aged 75 years and over. Not all patients in psychiatric hospitals who are aged 65 years and over, however, are 'psychogeriatric' cases; many will be 'graduate' patients, having reached the age of 65 years while resident long term in a mental illness hospital. About one-third of patients have been in hospital for at least 10 years.

Beds in Geriatric Hospitals

There were about 1600 people whose usual residence at the time of the 1981 Census was a geriatric hospital. The mean age of these patients was 81 years; 73 per cent were aged 75 years and over and 27 per cent were aged 85 years and over.

Of those resident in hospital on 31 December 1981, 29 per cent had been in hospital for less than 3 months, 25 per cent for 3–11 months, 21 per cent for 1–2 years, and 25 per cent for 3 years or more. The age breakdown of this resident population was 4 per cent under the age of 65 years, 9 per cent aged 65–69 years, 36 per cent aged 70–79 years, 42 per cent aged 80–89 years, and 9 per cent aged 90 years or over. Of those patients discharged or who died during 1981, 50 per cent were discharged home or to convalescent homes, 28 per cent died, 20 per cent were transferred to another hospital and 1·8 per cent were transferred to local authority care.

Analysis by area of usual residence of admissions to geriatric hospitals shows an approximately threefold variation in admission rates of the elderly between those 28 postcode sectors with the lowest rates and those 28 with the highest rates. The areas with the highest admission rates tend to be the more deprived areas of local authority housing and areas with a relatively high proportion of privately rented accomodation.

Residential Homes

The total number of places in residential homes available in the GGHB area in 1981 was 2800, of which 60 per cent were owned by local authorities, 35 per cent by voluntary organizations and only about 5 per cent were privately owned. By 1986 the number of private places had increased to about 8 per cent of the total. The age distribution of residents was very similar to that for geriatric hospitals except that there was a considerably greater proportion of people aged 90 years or above (12·3 per cent compared with 9 per cent in geriatric hospitals), and the mean age was slightly higher (82–83 years).

Sheltered Housing

There are some 104 sheltered housing complexes in the GGHB area, with a total of about 2500 places. Most are owned by the local authority, but increasing numbers are being built by housing associations and private building companies. No information is available centrally about the ages or health of people resident in sheltered housing.

Social Work Services

Table 2.2 gives the proportion of the population, aged 65 years and over and 75 years and over, which is in receipt of certain social work services in Glasgow City. The Table shows that the ratio of daily meals provided (at home or at a lunch club) to the population aged 75 years and over is 112 per 1000. However, considerably less than 10 per cent of the population in this age-group will receive such meals, because some will receive two or more meals each week, and many recipients will be under the age of 75 years. The proportion of people who receive the services of a home help will, however, be greater than 11·5 per cent (age 65 years and over) or 30 per cent (aged 75 years and over) (*see Table* 2.2) because many recipients will be couples rather than single individuals.

Table 2.2. Provision of home helps and meals

Service	*No.*	*No. per 1000 relevant population*	
		65+ yrs	*75+ yrs*
Home helps	13 784 (total caseload)	115	300
Home helps	2015 (FTEs)	17	44
Lunch clubs (local authority + voluntary	3656 (daily meals)	30	79
Meals on wheels	1513 (daily meals)	12.6	33
Population of Glasgow City		119 757	46 012

FTEs: Full–time equivalents.

Day Hospital Attendances

Table 2.3 gives annual attendance figures for geriatric day hospitals in the GGHB area, with rates for the population aged 65 years and over, and 75 years and over. This shows that only 0·19 per cent of the population aged 65 years and over attends a day hospital during any one year, and that on any one day the proportion is only 0·11 per cent. Day hospitals are on average less than 70 per cent occupied.

Table 2.3. Attendances at day hospitals

Day hospitals		*Rates per 1000 relevant population**	
	No.	*65+ yrs*	*75+ yrs*
Persons attending for first time in 1982–1983	2053	13·9	36·2
Total attendances during 1982–1983	40 040	271	706
Total persons attending at least once in 1982–1983	2782	18·8	49·1
Places available	243	1·6	4·3
Average daily attendance	167	1·1	2·9

* Based on 1982 mid-year population estimates for GGHB area.

The day hospitals work on different principles. The majority arrange attendances on one, two and sometimes three occasions each week for an indefinite period (which sometimes may extend to several years). Others organize short courses of treatment (e.g. for 8 weeks), after which the patient is usually discharged.

In a survey conducted during 1981 it was shown that the mean age of patients attending geriatric day hospitals was 81 years; 92 per cent of patients attended twice per week and 44 per cent of patients had attended for over 1 year.

Outpatient attendances

There are no psychogeriatric outpatient clinics in the GGHB area, nor are any data available about the numbers of elderly patients who attend ordinary psychiatric outpatient departments. *Table* 2.4, however, gives attendances at geriatric outpatient clinics.

Table 2.4. Attendances at geriatric outpatient clinics

Outpatient clinics		*Rates per 1000 relevant population**	
	No.	*65+ yrs*	*75+ yrs*
Persons attending for first time in 1981–1982	764	5·2	13·5
Total attendances during 1981–1982	3792	25·6	66·9

* Based on 1982 mid-year population estimates for GGHB area.

Summary of Available Residential Accomodation

The approximate number of available places within the GGHB area is given in *Table* 2.5 together with rates based on the population aged 65 years and over and aged 75 years and over. Also given in the Table for comparative purposes (in parentheses) are the rates of provision recommended in the Timbury (1979) and MacDonald (1980) reports.[1,2] The actual places available in the GGHB area approximate quite closely to these recommendations, although the distribution within the area is uneven.

Table 2.5. Summary of residential accommodation for the elderly within the GGHB area

Type of accommodation	*No. of beds/places**	*Beds/places per 1000 relevant population* 65+ *yrs*	75+ *yrs*
Sheltered housing (Housing)	2101	14·2 (25)	37·1
Residential homes (Social Work)	1947	18·9 (20)	49·3 }
(voluntary and private)	847		} 100
Geriatric Hospital (NHS)	2204	14·9 (15)	38·9 }
Psychogeriatric Hospital (NHS)	1685	11·4 (10)	29·7
Nursing Homes (Private)	310	2·1	5·5
GGHB population†			
65+ years	148 012	—	—
75+ years	56 692	—	—

* As in 1982.
† 1981 mid-year estimate.
Figures in parentheses give recommended numbers of beds/places.

COMMUNITY NURSING

The decennial census, conducted in April 1981, provided an opportunity to determine the proportion of the elderly population in receipt of community nursing services—in total, in broad age/sex groupings and according to whether the client was living alone or with others. On a single day during the first fortnight of September 1981 a census was therefore conducted of all elderly clients on the current caseload of health visitors or district nurses employed by the GGHB.

Table 2.6 gives the total number of GGHB residents (including those normally resident in institutions), by sex and 5-year age-groups, together with the number and proportion in those groups currently on the caseload of health visitors and district nurses. About 9 per cent of the elderly (aged 65 years and over) are on the health visitors' caseload, and about 4·3 per cent are currently receiving treatment from the district nurses. There is, however, a marked gradation with age. For example, only 2·6 per cent of those in the 65–69-year age-group are on the health visitors' caseload whereas 24 per cent of those in the oldest (85 years and over) age-group are so included. The corresponding figures for the district nurses are 1·4 and 15·4 per cent.

Table 2.6. Elderly persons currently on the caseload of health visitors and district nurses

Age-group (yrs)	*Population (all residents)**	*Health visitors*		*District nurses*	
		No. on caseload	*% on caseload*	*No. on caseload*	*% on caseload*
Men					
65–69	21 497	377	1·7	205	0·95
70–74	16 314	769	4·7	319	2·0
75–79	9745	907	9·3	366	3·8
80–84	4090	650	15·9	270	6·6
85+	1792	406	22·7	220	12·3
N/K	—	110	—	13	—
Total	53 438	3219	6·0	1393	2·6
Women					
65–69	28 554	947	3·3	486	1·7
70–74	25 095	2002	8·0	784	3·1
75–79	19 258	2658	13·8	1130	5·9
80–84	11 623	2459	21·2	1185	10·2
85+	6991	1710	24·5	1132	16·2
N/K	—	345	—	47	—
Total	91 521	10 121	11·1	4764	5·2
Total					
65–69	50 051	1325	2·6	692	1·4
70–74	41 409	2773	6·7	1105	2·7
75–79	29 003	3568	12·3	1499	5·2
80–84	15 713	3110	19·8	1457	9·3
85+	8783	2107	24·0	1354	15·4
N/K	—	456	—	62	—
Total	144 959	13 339	9·2	6169	4·3

* Mid-year estimate, 30 June 1981 (1981 Census based). N/K = not known.

There is considerable difference between the sexes: in the younger age-group (65–74 years) women are almost twice as likely as men to be under the care or surveillance of a health visitor or district nurse, and this tendency is repeated—although to a lesser extent—in the older age-groups. *Table* 2.6 also shows that the 5-year age-groups from which most clients are derived (for both the health visitors and district nurses) are the 75–79-year age-group of men, and the 75–79 and 80–84-year age-groups of women. Sixty-four per cent of the health visitors' and 60 per cent of the district nurses' caseload of elderly were aged 75 years or over. The corresponding figures for the age-group 80 years and over are 38 and 48 per cent.

The investigation also showed that for the GGHB area as a whole, elderly people who lived alone were almost twice as likely to be visited in the past year by a health visitor or support staff as people who live with others for district nursing, however, the difference was considerably less. Of those living alone, 15 per cent aged 65 years and over and 25 per cent of those aged 75 years and over had been visited by the health visitor or support staff during the previous 12 months; the corresponding figures for those currently on the district nurses' caseload were 6 and 10 per cent.

Further analysis demonstrated an almost sixfold difference in the proportion of elderly on the health visitors' caseload between the 20 per cent of the GGHB population living in the areas with the highest rates for health visiting, and the 20 per cent living in the areas with the lowest rates. The differences in the proportion of elderly on the district nurses' caseload were considerably smaller—the difference between the highest and lowest 20 per cent of the population being a factor of two. Some areas with the lowest health visiting and district nursing rates were in the most disadvantaged communities. There was no evidence that areas with relatively low caseloads for one service compensate by having relatively high caseloads for the other; if anything the opposite is true.

A similar type of analysis was conducted of the proportion of those receiving support from community nursing staff (both health visitors and district nurses) who were in addition reported as receiving support from home helps, chiropodists and occupational therapists. These analyses demonstrated a threefold geographic variation between the areas in the lowest and highest quintiles for home help and chiropody services, and almost a sixfold difference for occupational therapy services.

In view of the considerable differences in utilization of services, particularly in relation to health visitors, it would be interesting to assess how surveillance actually benefits the client. Is there, for example, any demographic difference between elderly people living in areas where health visiting rates are higher and those living in areas where rates are low? Is any measurable benefit derived by the elderly who live in areas with relatively high health visiting rates? How are the elderly selected for visiting by health visitors, and are they the ones who are most in need?. What is the relationship between the health visitor and other serivces such as home helps, and to what extent do they compensate for one another? What form of intervention by the health visitor is of greatest benefit—is it by helping to obtain support from other agencies, by the early detection of medical problems, or simply by providing an opportunity for old people to talk things over?

SPATIAL VARIATION IN DEATH RATES OF THE ELDERLY

The availability of age-specific population data for 1981 by postcode sector of residence provided the opportunity for calculating mortality rates for relatively small areas within the health authority. Rates were calculated for both sexes in combination for each of the age-groups

15–59 years, 60–64, 65–69, 70–74, 75–79, 80–84 and 85 years and over. The rates for the 15–59-year age-group were standardized for age and sex. The difference in the mean death rate for the 28 postcode sectors in the quintile with the highest rates and the 28 postcode sectors in the quintile with the lowest rates was 2·5-fold for the 15–59-year age-group, just over twofold in the 60–64 age-group, just under twofold in each of the four 65–84 age-groups, but only 1·2-fold in the age-group 85 years and over. This means that for people over the entire age-range 60–84 years, residents of the 'higher' quintile of postcode sectors have about twice the likelihood of dying in any one year compared with residents of areas in the 'lowest' quintile. Each of the major causes of death (ischaemic heart disease, malignant disease and cerebrovascular disease) contributed to these differences. There was marked consistency between the various age-groups in the mortality rating for the postcode sectors, the postcode sectors with the highest death rates being located entirely in the more disadvantaged areas of the city and suburbs.

It is evident, therefore, that those who reside in areas with high death rates and reach pensionable age still have a reduced expectation of life compared with those who live in areas with low death rates.

Table 2.7 illustrates the socioeconomic characteristics of the total population in those quintiles with the lowest and highest death rates with reference to five indicators derived from the 1981 Census. The extreme difference between the two types of area is evident from the Table. The postcode sectors with the highest mortality rates have on average five times the rate of unemployment among men, over five times the proportion of the population in social classes IV and V, about four times the proportion of local authority housing and of overcrowded households, and three times the prevalence of children living in single-parent households.

Table 2.7. Socioeconomic characteristics of the population resident in the postcode sectors in the highest and lowest quintiles of mortality, Census 1981

	Mortality rating	
Census indicator	*Highest quintile*	*Lowest quintile*
% children <16 yrs living in single-parent households	26·0 (22·7–51·8)	6·0 (0·2–7·1)
% unemployed men (16–64 yrs)	30·8 (19·2–45·9)	6·1 (3·3–15·3)
% housing owned by local authority	72·7 (18·3–96·2)	17·4 (0·1–48·5)
% overcrowded households*	26·2 (17·2–41·1)	7·7 (2·6–17·5)
% population in social classes IV and V	43·5 (8·0–84·0)	7·9 (2·0–15·0)

Figures in parentheses indicate the ranges for the 22 postcode sectors in each quintile.
* Defined as more than one person per room.

INVESTIGATION OF DISCHARGES OF ELDERLY PATIENTS FROM MEDICAL WARDS AT GLASGOW ROYAL INFIRMARY

In 1982 a research health visitor was employed to follow up, over a 39-week period, all patients in the acute medical wards of Glasgow Royal Infirmary who were declared medically fit for discharge. Patients were deemed to have had an 'excess' stay if they remained in hospital for longer than 7 days after being declared medically fit for discharge.

Of 140 patients so identified, 75 eventually received their recommended placement. Nineteen died while awaiting placement, 22 continued to 'block' an acute bed and 24 received alternative placements.

About two-thirds of the 84 patients who were recommended for accommodation in a geriatric hospital received this placement; for 11 of those who were not placed, the geriatric hospital appropriate to their usual residence was situated in a neighbouring health authority, and none of these patients was in fact admitted during the survey. Of 12 patients recommended for accommodation in a psychogeriatric hospital only 1 was admitted. Of 7 recommended for a residential home 3 were admitted, and of 9 recommended for a hospice again only 3 were admitted.

In all, the acute medical beds were 'blocked' for a total of 6740 days during the survey—equivalent to 18·5 permanently occupied beds or about 20 per cent of the total occupied bed days for these wards.

A follow-up study was conducted at 4 and at 12 weeks of the 35 patients who were discharged home after an 'excess' stay in hospital. Of these discharges 19 were planned (home having been the recommended placement) and 16 were unplanned—the latter group usually being sent home with less than 48 hours' notice in order to free beds for use by others.

Of the 19 planned discharges home, 14 had been delayed while waiting for home help services (4 were also awaiting day hospital or day centre care) and in 5 cases there was difficulty in arranging help from relatives. Of the 16 unplanned discharges, 13 had been waiting for hospital placement, 2 for hospice provision and 1 had been waiting for a place in a convalescent home.

Twelve weeks after discharge, 13 of the 19 patients whose discharge home had been planned were still at home, although only 8 of these were considered to be coping adequately. The remaining 6 patients had been readmitted to hospital, and of these 3 had died. Of the 16 patients whose discharge home had not been planned, only 8 were still living at home after 12 weeks, and of these only 2 were regarded as coping reasonably well, 2 coping with considerable difficulty, and 4 were living in an extremely unsatisfactory situation with marked physical and/or mental deterioration. The remaining 8 patients in this group had all been readmitted to hospital, and 3 of these had died.

The following recommendations were made as a result of this study:

1. Full assessment of self-care ability, of domestic support available, and provision of a social report should be mandatory for all elderly patients prior to discharge.
2. The arrangement of supportive community services on discharge should be more effectively coordinated, including greater involvement of the primary care team.
3. A full-time liaison nurse should be appointed to deal with the needs of the elderly in this one hospital. The current inadequate social work provision is directed mainly to the needs of wage-earners. The liaison nurse would be the 'key worker' to the elderly, would coordinate arrangements for transfer or discharge, and would assess the adequacy of the support services.
4. Geriatric catchment areas should be organized so that geriatric long-stay accommodation is available locally and is certainly not the responsibility of another health authority.
5. There should be investigation of reasons for the permanent overcrowding of psychogeriatric beds when provision within the GGHB area exceeds the recommended norm. This may, for example, be due to the misplacement of patients or to lack of availability of caring relatives.
6. Improvement in communication between geriatricians and physicians is required, with a consultant geriatrician possibly becoming a member of the medical team in acute medical wards.
7. Consideration should be given to establishing augmented home care for the elderly in their own homes when they develop an acute illness not necessitating admission to hospital, or to the provision of community geriatric teams incorporating the services and resources of the local geriatrician and his or her staff in addition to the primary care teams.

CHANGES WITH AGE IN THE USE OF HEALTH SERVICES

Over the period 1986–2001 the numbers of elderly in the population will remain approximately constant, or even decline slightly. This projection, however, disguises marked differences between the various age-groups: the numbers in the age-group 65–74 years will decline by about 8 per cent, whereas those for the 75–84-year and 85-years and over age-groups will increase by respectively about 8 and 55 per cent. After the age of 65 years there is an approximately linear increase on a logarithmic scale in the use of services: at age 85 years the proportion of the population resident in an institution or receiving the services of a home help is about 10 times that for the population aged 65 years; the corresponding difference in the death rate or for inpatient day stay in hospital is about fivefold.[3]

The less numerous but rapidly increasing older age-groups within the population aged 65 years and over therefore make much bigger demands on health and social services than the younger (65–74 years) age-group. Thus, although the absolute number of people aged 65 years and over will decrease over the next 15 years, the demands on health and social services will increase because of the increased number of the very elderly: this increase is likely to be in the range 25–60 per cent.[3]

SOME CONCLUSIONS FROM OUR INFORMATION SOURCES

1. The proportion of elderly in the population shows considerable geographical variation, and there are considerable differences in housing conditions—from spacious accommodation in owner-occupied housing in pleasant residential areas to overcrowded accommodation in privately rented or local authority housing in less attractive areas.

2. The proportion of old people who normally live in institutions (mainly old persons' homes and psychiatric and geriatric hospitals) varies from 2·4 per cent in the 65–74-year age-group to 20·4 per cent in those aged 85 years and over.

3. People aged 65 years and over occupy almost 50 per cent of acute hospital beds.

4. No information is collated centrally about the characteristics of old people in residential accommodation, in sheltered housing, who 'block' acute beds, who receive home helps or meals on wheels, or who attend day hospitals or lunch clubs.

5. The number of places in residential homes and geriatric hospitals within the Glasgow area is only slightly below national recommendations.

6. The proportion of elderly people on the caseload of a health visitor varies widely within the GGHB area, and many of the most disadvantaged areas have the smallest proportions. There is a similar variation in the utilization of home helps, chiropody and—to a lesser extent—district nursing services, and again the disadvantaged areas often have the lowest utilization rates.

7. The role of the health visitor in relation to the elderly has not been clearly defined. It may be as a 'key worker' in coordinating the help of the agencies, for the detection of previously unknown medical problems or simply for providing occasional social contact.

8. The death rate of the elderly who live in the more disadvantaged areas is approximately twice that of those who live in the more affluent areas.

9. On average 20 per cent of the acute medical beds at one major hospital are permanently occupied by elderly patients who no longer require acute medical care. The main reasons for this relate to

difficulties in providing hospital accommodation for psychogeriatric patients and to differences in the catchment areas for acute and geriatric populations. In comparison, there was relatively little difficulty in providing community support services. Major difficulties are, however, caused by elderly patients being discharged home, often with little notice, when their recommended placement is a hospital (geriatric or psychogeriatric), residential home or hospice.

10. Admission rates to acute and geriatric hospitals are greater, by a factor of two or three in the more deprived inner-city areas, in the peripheral housing schemes and in the areas of relatively high proportions of privately rented accommodation compared with the more affluent parts of the Glasgow area.

INFORMATION AS A BASE FOR PLANNING

At present, at least in the Glasgow area, information is used to a minimal extent in managing or planning services for the elderly. There are thus many inequalities and other deficiencies in the way that services are organized, of which the following are some examples:

1. There is no uniform system for selection of patients for inclusion in the health visitors' caseload; in some areas there is a systematic attempt to visit all patients, using an age/sex register as a means of identification, whereas elsewhere the health visitor may only visit patients referred by other health personnel or by other agencies. As a result some health visitors have relatively large numbers of elderly people on their caseload, whereas others have very few. It has been suggested that most energy should be devoted to managing the problems (acute and chronic disease) that elderly people present, and that if we were to develop a more systematic approach to clinical practice we should concentrate our efforts on better management of chronic diseases than on an elaborate programme of case finding.[4] In view of the many problems identified in services for the elderly in Glasgow it would seem reasonable to adopt this policy, rather than to dissipate efforts in case finding that is of unproven value.

2. No attempt has been made to target service provision on geographical areas where the elderly have particularly high mortality and admission rates. These are in general the areas with the poorest housing and socioeconomic circumstances.

3. Despite the fact that almost 50 per cent of acute hospital beds are occupied by patients over the age of 65 years, there is little effective collaboration between the medical staff in these hospitals and geriatricians in the assessment of patients prior to discharge. Also, there appears to be no organizational mechanism available for finding alternative suitable placements when the geriatric or psychogeriatric

hospital appropriate to the patient's home is unable or unwilling to provide accommodation, nor has it been possible to resolve the problem of catchment areas that extend into adjacent authorities or to determine why psychogeriatric hospital accommodation is severely 'blocked' when bed provision approximates to the recommended norms.

4. The link between acute medical and community services is still unsatisfactory, usually being delegated, often too late, to relatively junior hospital staff. There is no system of monitoring the adequacy of provision of services in the community nor of feedback of such information to hospital staff. Some structured assessment of capabilities and community and social support is required prior to discharge from hospital, and active involvement of the primary care team is required prior to and after discharge. The appointment of liaison nurses, and the establishment of community geriatric teams or of augmented home care for the elderly are other solutions that require consideration.

PLANNING SERVICES FOR THE ELDERLY

Although services for the elderly have been designated high priority,[5] little progress has been made in diverting resources from the acute sector and relatively little improvement in services has been achieved. One stimulus for progress may be the recent Scottish Office circular *Community Care: Joint Planning and Support Finance*.[6] The circular stresses the importance of close cooperation between local authority, health services, voluntary and other agencies to ensure the efficient use of their resources in meeting the needs of particular client groups. It requires local authorities and health authorities to draw up joint plans that concentrate on priority categories identified in the SHAPE report.[5] Specifically, the circular recommends that the joint plans should:

1. Assess the need for the provision of services for priority categories.
2. Set out the main objectives to be achieved in the next 10 years.
3. Take account of the resources available.
4. Quantify the effects of the plans' objectives on expenditure, hospital beds, health and local authority service provision, etc.

It is to be hoped that the need to formulate such joint plans will bring the needs of particular client groups, including the elderly, into focus and will lead to the formulation of targets and of methods of monitoring performance in relation to these objectives.

CONCLUSION

Despite the clear demonstration of many inadequacies in the care of the elderly, little progress has been made towards the resolution of these difficulties. Part of the reason for this is the relative lack of effective pressure groups such as exist in the fields of maternal and child health. Other reasons are lack of interest among professionals, and the absence of hard indices against which performance may be measured. Health and local authorities are, however, now being required to formulate joint plans and to set specific objectives for the care of individual client groups and to demonstrate the extent to which these are being achieved. It is hoped that this will provide the necessary impetus to bring about a substantial improvement over the next 10 years in the provision of well-coordinated health and social services for the elderly.

REFERENCES

1. Timbury G. C. (1979) *Report on Services for the Elderly with Mental Disability in Scotland.* Scottish Home and Health Department and Scottish Education Department. Edinburgh, SHHD HMSO.
2. MacDonald Elizabeth (1980) *Changing Patterns of Care.* Scottish Education Department. Edinburgh, SHHD HMSO.
3. Craig J. (1983) *Popul. Trends.* (1983) **32**, 28.
4. Dr Stringfellow's Team (1986) Prevention for patients over 75: is it worth the bother? *Br. Med. J.* **ii**, 1243.
5. SHAPE (1980) *Scottish Health Authorities Priorities for the Eighties.* Edinburgh, HMSO.
6. Scottish Home and Health Department (1985) *Community Care: Joint Planning and Support Finance.* SHHD Circular NHS 1985 (GEN) 18. Edinburgh, HMSO.

3. GERIATRIC CARE IN A RURAL SETTING

D. R. Hannay

Wigtownshire lies in the extreme southwest of Southwest Scotland and is one of the four administrative districts of the Dumfries and Galloway region. (*Fig.* 3.1) It is a rural area with a population of approximately 29 000. There are two centres of population—Stranraer and Newton Stewart. The former is a ferry terminal for the Northern Ireland crossing and has a population of about 10 000, while the latter is a market town with a population of about 4000.

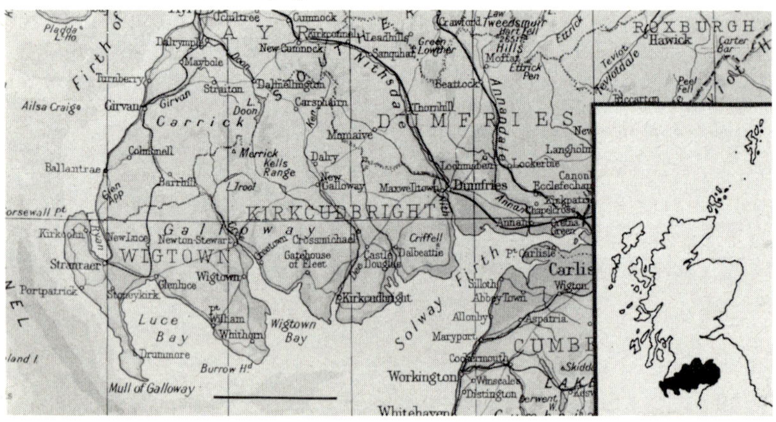

Fig. 3.1. Map of Southwest Scotland showing Wigtownshire, Kirkcudbrightshire and Dumfriesshire. Horizontal bar = 32 km. *Inset* shows Galloway in relation to Scotland.

Like many such areas there is a high proportion of elderly people. This is partly because of rural depopulation, with the decline in jobs on the land being reflected in high unemployment figures especially among school leavers. As the young go away to seek work elsewhere, so the proportion of elderly in the population rises. A lower birth rate for those who remain increases this tendency, as does the number of people retiring to the area. The boom in caravan sites and second homes has tailed off in recent years, but more people have become aware of the attractions of Galloway, although expanding tourism has not resulted in sufficient employment to offset rural depopulation.

In a sense there are two phases of retirement, especially for those coming into the area from outside. For the first 10 years or so after 65, an elderly couple can enjoy their chosen home in the country with activities such as gardening and other outdoor pursuits. However, after 75 the afflictions of old age reduce mobility and increase dependence especially if one partner dies. There may then be another move to be with grown-up children, who are usually working in or near a conurbation. If this is not feasible then caring services in the rural area are increasingly called on.

In the last Census 18 per cent of the population in Wigtownshire were of pensionable age compared to 16·8 per cent for Scotland as a whole. This represented an 11·2 per cent increase for the area over the decade since the previous Census, compared to an 8·7 per cent increase for Scotland as a whole. Those aged 75 years and over make up 5·7 per cent of the population of Wigtownshire compared with 5·3 per cent for Scotland, and for this age-group the intercensal increase for Wigtownshire was 30·6 per cent—the largest for any district in Scotland. For Dumfries and Galloway region as a whole it is estimated that the number of over-75s will increase by 24 per cent between 1981 and 1990, whereas the total population of the region will rise by only 0·8 per cent over the same period.

The implications of these demographic changes for the provision of services for the elderly are considerable. In many respects the district is well served, but its geography makes special demands on the different kinds of services required for an ageing population. These services are now considered in terms of community care, residential care and hospital care with special reference to the latter in a rural area.

COMMUNITY CARE

Community care is provided by general practitioners, nurses, social workers and other professional groups such as domiciliary physiotherapists and chiropodists. In addition there is special housing and a range of voluntary services. General practitioners in Galloway tend to have below-average list sizes, and some are dispensing practices with a considerable amount of rural mileage payments. The community nursing services are well developed with practice attachments, and together with physiotherapy departments the community nurses are responsible for a range of home care equipment. Expensive adaptations to the home require financial approval from the social work department, and this can cause administrative delays. About 350 people in the district are getting approximately 6·5 hours per person per week of home help, and 170 people receive meals on wheels for 3 days a week distributed by the WRVS. There is a need for more domiciliary physiotherapy services, and there are known to be a number of unemployed physiotherapists in the area seeking work. There are also long waiting lists for chiropody services in spite of a mobile unit for rural areas and a laundry service would greatly help the families of those being nursed at home.

There are 72 sheltered housing units in the district provided by the local authority and Kirk Care. More are planned and needed. The social work department is due to install a community alarm system in Stranraer by which any house can be linked for emergency services to a central warden. Such a system could profitably be extended throughout the district, especially to more isolated rural areas, rather than just in the town as envisaged at present.

There are a number of strong voluntary organizations that provide invaluable services to the elderly. As well as meals on wheels the WRVS runs a clothes service, transport service and visiting service for those confined to their home. The Red Cross is also active in providing transport and home visiting, among other activities. There are a number of fund-raising organizations such as the Hospital Volunteer Committees, and Crossroads has recently started in the district, financed by the Manpower Services Commission.

RESIDENTIAL CARE

Residential care is provided by Part IV accommodation, to which about 30 people are admitted each year in the Wigtown district, with about half that number again for holiday admissions. Additional beds are being provided, and the health criteria for admission are becoming less rigid, with priority being given to hospital patients. Increasingly those in Part IV accommodation require some form of nursing care, and specific community nurses are being assigned for this task.

HOSPITAL CARE

The main district general hospital is in Dumfries about 80 km away, but there are two local hospitals in Stranraer and one in Newton Stewart. One of the Stranraer hospitals has 44 beds, of which 20 are general practitioner and 24 surgical beds under a consultant surgeon. Every winter a high proportion of these is blocked by long-stay patients. The other hospital in Stranraer has 48 geriatric beds, a few of which are occupied by young chronic sick, and 5 are used as holiday beds on a fortnightly basis.

The only other hospital provision is in Newton Stewart where the local hospital has 27 beds, 9 of which are general practitioner beds, and the remainder long-stay beds under consultant geriatricians. Whereas in Stranraer the geriatric beds are looked after by one of the general practitioners, who has a sessional appointment with consultant cover, in Newton Stewart all the patients, whether in general practitioner or long-stay beds, are looked after by their own doctor. This has resulted in a more active use of the beds, as family doctors are aware of home circumstances and can more easily make arrangements for periods at home or in hospital.

Another important factor in the use of the Newton Stewart hospital beds has been the advent of the day hospital, which was started in 1979 with 1 day a week, and now functions for 5 days a week with the help of equipment provided by the hospital's League of Friends. As the facilities of the day hospital expanded, so the turnover in beds increased with more short-stay holiday admissions in general practitioner beds. An increase in discharge from the long-stay beds also became possible with day hospital support for patients being cared for at home.

The effect of the day hospital on bed turnover in Newton Stewart is shown in *Table* 3.1. The hospital's League of Friends was started in 1977 and provided transport for the day hospital. As these facilities increased so did the turnover of hospital beds, until the past 2 or 3 years, when an increasingly elderly population has put such pressure on the day hospital that there is no longer a continuing increase in bed turnover. For the long-stay beds a recent decrease in admissions and discharges is partly due to a decline in the number of deaths. But overall the impact of the day hospital with the active involvement of general practitioners looking after their own patients, has been to increase dramatically the use of beds in Newton Stewart hospital. This contrasts with the 48-bed hospital in Stranraer which in 1984 had 124 admissions, compared to 178 admissions to the 27-bed hospital in Newton Stewart.

Table 3.1. Day hospital provision and use of beds in Newton Stewart Hospital

	1976	*1977*	*1978*	*1979*	*1980*	*1981*	*1982*	*1983*	*1984*
Day hospital (days per week)	0	0	0	1	2	2	2	3	5
Admissions per year to 9 GP beds	44	63	63	50	42	75	108	114	146
Admissions per year to 18 long-stay beds	4	17	17	11	24	30	35	37	32
Holiday beds		Occasional in summer				2 all year		3 all year	

Over the past year or so the turnover of hospital beds has not been able to keep pace with the requirements of an increasingly elderly population, and there is an urgent need for more beds. In 1986 there were 18 patients blocking hospital beds in Dumfries over 80 km away, and many more being supported in the community by the day hospital and holiday admissions, who could need long-stay beds at any time. One of the local general practices calculated that the lack of beds in Newton Stewart hospital resulted in 20 ambulance trips over a period of 6 months to Dumfries or back. This amounts to about 1600 km of ambulance journeys per year. Quite apart from the cost of this, the distress and hardship to patients and relatives in rural areas who have to travel at least 80 km to the nearest hospital in Dumfries are considerable.

If existing provisions are inadequate now they will be more so in the future. Much has been done for the elderly with existing community services, but in rural areas there is a need for more domiciliary services such as chiropody and physiotherapy, as well as sheltered housing. But the main requirement is for hospital beds under general practitioner care in the local community. As has been shown in Newton Stewart much can be done with the limited resources and the imaginative use of day hospital facilities and cooperation with Part IV accommodation. But the increased proportion of elderly people necessitates a realistic provision of hospital beds in the local community both for long-stay patients and to provide holiday relief for the rising number of geriatric patients being maintained in their own homes.

A further important factor in the future care of the elderly is the ability of general practitioners to use microcomputers to monitor their practice populations. It is now possible in the West of Scotland for practice age–sex registers to be made available on floppy discs from a central mainframe computer, which stores the primary care data for a number of health boards. Software is available to enable general practitioners to monitor repeat prescriptions, problem lists and nursing care among other factors. It is therefore possible to provide anticipatory care for the elderly rather than just to react to events.

4. FAVOURABLE DEMOGRAPHIC ASPECTS OF THE ELDERLY FOR THE NEXT 30 YEARS

F. I. Caird

In the United Kingdom the principal demographic change in the next 30 years will be an inescapable rise in the numbers of very old people whose much greater needs for health care[1,2] will impose a further considerable load on caring agencies of all kinds. This increase in the numbers of the elderly is both in absolute and even more in relative terms, because the decline in the birth rate since the turn of the century also entails a reduction in the numbers of younger people to care for the elderly.

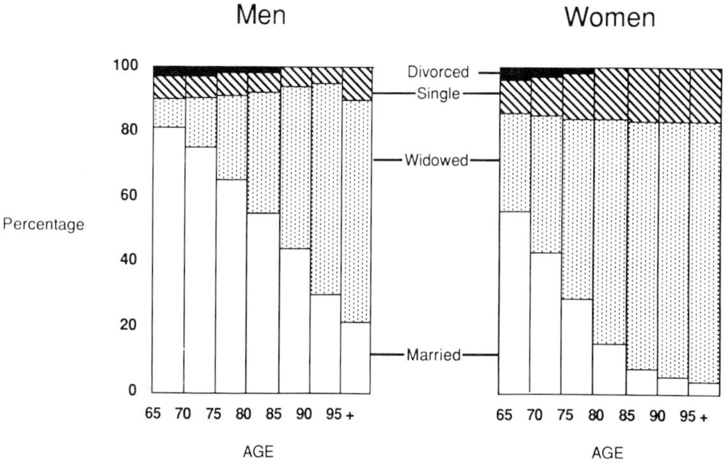

Fig. 4.1. Proportions of elderly people in Great Britain by marital status and age at 1981 Census. *Source*: OPCS (1983) *1981 Census*. London, HMSO.

A convenient starting point for a discussion of the demographic factors involved is the situation of the elderly at the 1981 Census (*Fig.* 4.1). There is a substantial increase with age in the proportion of widowers and widows (particularly the latter) and a concomitant decline in the numbers of those of both sexes still married. The proportion of single persons increases, by about half, from the age of

65 to that of 95 and over, from 10 to 16 per cent in women and from 8 to 12 per cent in men. The proportion of old people who are at this time divorced is so small as to be almost negligible; it is only 2–3 per cent at the age of 65, and falls to 0·4 per cent at most over the age of 95. The figures as given refer to those single, divorced, married or widowed at the time of the Census, and thus do not distinguish between those married only once and those married more than once. This proportion will doubtless increase with time, maybe substantially so, as divorce becomes more common. Marriage more than once does not necessarily imply the benefit to be expected from the acquisition of two families, either or even both of which are, in theory at least, available to support their elderly parents. There is much anecdotal evidence from geriatricians that elderly men who have married twice may succeed in alienating both families, and so be as disadvantaged in this respect as those who have remained single. Maybe there is a moral here, particularly for men.

The major demographic factors relevant for the future are all operative now, and all are subject to considerable secular trends. They are four in number: the marriage rate, family size and composition, the differential mortality of the sexes, and population mobility. There is one important difference between the first two of these and the last two. The first two cannot change or be manipulated in any way, since they have already happened. The differential mortality between the sexes can certainly change in future years but is very difficult to manipulate. Population mobility can be manipulated up to a point by inducements by local and central government, but the relevant decisions require the difficult matters of an act of will on the part of politicians in power, and the ability to carry through what has been decided.

MARRIAGE RATE

The two main demographically demonstrable determinants of the requirement for institutional care, whether local authority or in nursing homes or (to a lesser extent) in hospital, have long been known to be age itself and the unmarried state. The importance of age in this context is shown by figures for Leicestershire,[4] which demonstrate that the rate of local authority institutional care doubles for both sexes approximately every 6 years over the age of 65 (*Fig*. 4.2), so that it is 25 times greater over the age of 90 than at 65–74. The much greater numbers of the 'younger' elderly mean that they provide most of the clients (*Fig*. 4.3). The second is illustrated by the fact that single old people of either sex are twice as likely to be in local authority institutional care as the widowed of the same age. At age 85 and over, they are approximately 10 times as likely to be in care as those who are still married (*Table* 4.1).

Table 4.1. Local authority institutional care: residence rates per 1000 population by marital status, age and sex[5]

	Present age (yrs)				
	60–64	*65–74*	*75–84*	*85+*	*Total 65+*
Male					
Married	—	—	—	17	1
Widowed/divorced	5	19	45	109	39
Single	11	39	105	253	66
Female					
Married	—	—	3	27	1
Widowed/divorced	1	5	27	95	21
Single	5	13	52	191	37

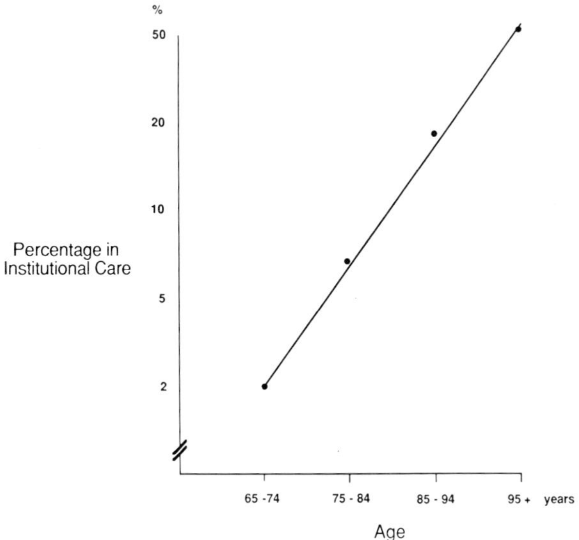

Fig. 4.2. Proportion of elderly people in Leicestershire in local authority residential care by age. *Source*: Donaldson L. J., Clarke M. and Palmer R. L. (1983) *Health Trends* **15**, 58.

Nothing direct can be done about age, but it follows that any change in the marriage rate in the lifetime of the future generation of the elderly may influence the requirement for institutional care. That such a change has already occurred is shown by the increasing proportion of single people over the age of 65 mentioned above and illustrated in *Fig.* 4.1. The implication is that the present 65-year-olds, as they age, will reduce the proportion of the single elderly by a not inconsiderable amount—an undoubtedly favourable factor.

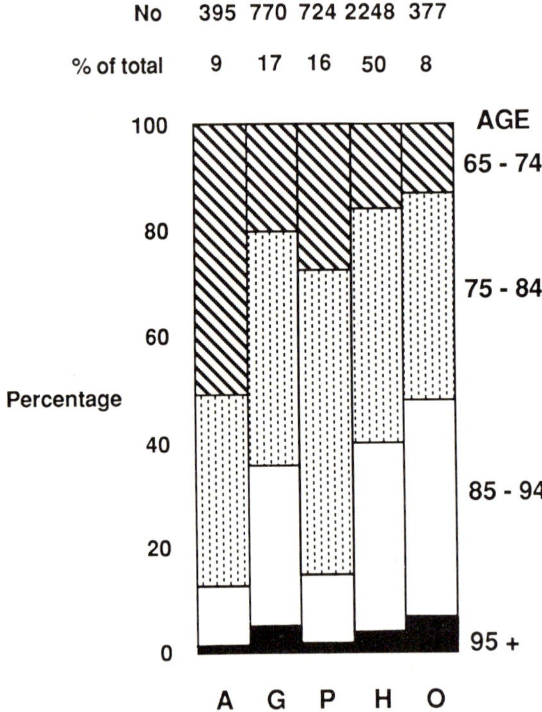

Fig. 4.3. Numbers and proportions by age of the elderly in Leicestershire in institutions. A, Acute hospitals; G, Geriatric hospitals; P, Psychiatric hospitals; H, Homes for the elderly; O, Other. *Source*: Donaldson L. J., Clarke M. and Palmer R. L. (1983) *Health Trends* **15**, 58.

FAMILY SIZE AND COMPOSITION

The decline in the mean size of the completed family since the beginning of the century is illustrated in *Fig.* 4.4. Women born in 1870 (and therefore at their median age of childbirth of 28 in 1898) had a mean size of completed family of 3·4. This fell to approximately 1·8 for those born in the early years of this century, and has fluctuated between 2·0 and 2·4 for those born in the middle of this century. This overall decline in family size certainly reduces the numbers of old

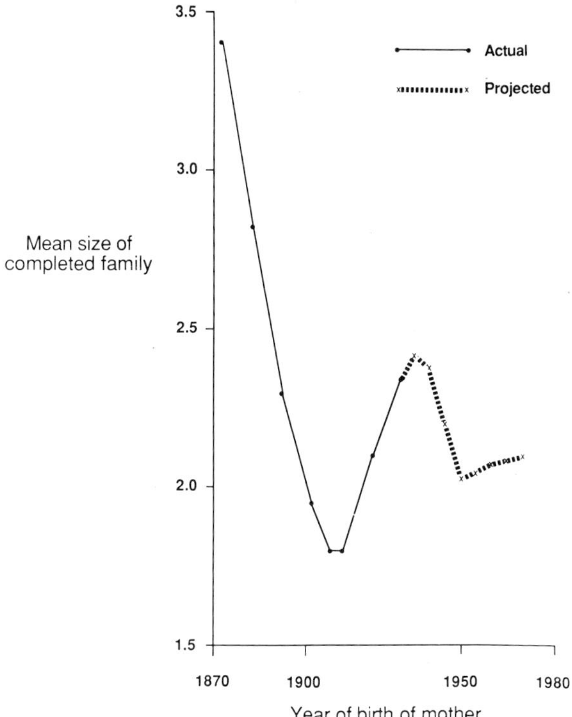

Fig. 4.4. Mean size of completed family in England and Wales, by year of birth of mother, 1870–1970. *Source*: OPCS (1981) *Population Projections 1978–2018* PP2 No. 10. London, HMSO, Table 7b.

people, whether married, widowed or single, who are available to provide support for their elderly siblings. This support is particularly important in respect of the single. In one study in Glasgow,[7] which is probably not unrepresentative on this point, nearly half of all single old people lived with a sibling. Forty-two per cent were visited at least once a week by a sibling; the commonsense view is that this is also a measure of support, albeit crude.

This dramatic fall in the mean size of the completed family conceals the important fact that the composition of families has changed over time, in that the proportion of childless marriages has fallen from 20 to 15 per cent or even at times to 10 per cent, while at the same time the proportion with two children has increased substantially, from 27 to 48 per cent (*Fig*. 4.5). There will, therefore, and somewhat paradoxically, be a greater proportion of married and widowed old people who have children to support them, and children are of course the principal support of the elderly. This is therefore a second favourable demographic factor for the future.

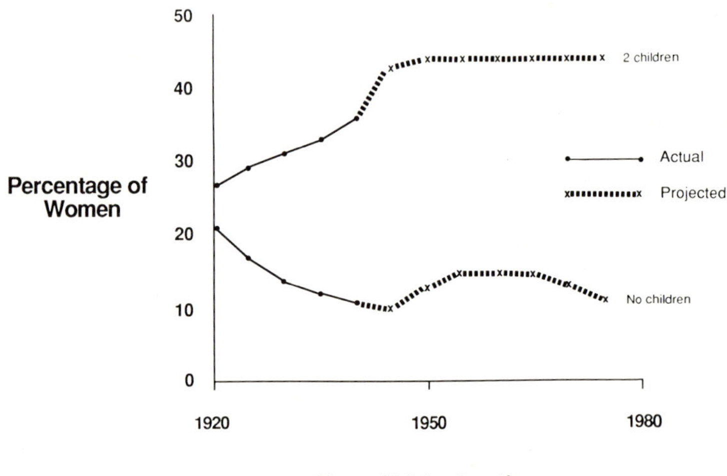

Fig. 4.5. Percentage of women in England and Wales with no and two children, by year of birth of mother, 1920–1970. *Source*: OPCS (1985) *Population Projections 1983–2023*. PP2 No. 13. London, HMSO, Appdx Table 3A1.

DIFFERENTIAL MORTALITY BY SEX

The differing mortality of the sexes in old age is shown by their differing expectations of life (*see* Chapter 5). The mortality of men is one principal cause of there being, age for age, a much greater proportion of widows than widowers in the elderly population, as shown in *Fig*. 4.1. The second is the fact that on average men marry women younger than themselves so that their wives are less far advanced along the relationship between age and mortality.

It is difficult to envisage that the latter of these two factors will change greatly, or that in the immediate future there will be either an increase in the expectation of life of elderly men, or a decrease in that of women, or both. However, the changes in the pattern of cigarette smoking that have taken place in recent years, with a decrease in smoking by men and an increase in that by younger and middle-aged women, would be expected to have this effect in the longer term. This would constitute a favourable factor for men but not for women.

Other potential changes in disease pattern (e.g. an improvement in mortality from carcinoma of the breast resulting from effective screening) would also affect differential mortality, but the consequences of the totality of such changes are impossible to predict with sufficient certainty to be of any value.

POPULATION MOBILITY

Population mobility is, as has been stated, an aspect of demography that can perhaps be altered in ways beneficial to the elderly. The very considerable extent of geographical mobility in the children of the elderly is shown by the Glasgow study previously mentioned.[7] In this, although 63 per cent of those with children had a child at least within a distance that made a day visit possible, as many as 10 per cent of all children lived overseas, and 27 per cent were outside Scotland but still within the United Kingdom. The study may not on this point be entirely representative of the country as a whole, since emigration has been a major feature of Scottish demography for at least two centuries. Nevertheless, the mobility of younger people in the country as a whole is also large. Its consequences can be manipulated in respect of the care of the elderly by a housing policy that actively encourages old people to move near to their children (and theoretically also vice versa). This has been the policy operated by several Scottish new towns, and although it has not been entirely successful in that a not insignificant proportion of elderly people prefer to return to where they were born and brought up, and do in fact do so, at least some contribution is made to the care of the elderly in the sense that more are in their own homes near their families, who are thus better placed to contribute to their support. The deliberate pursuit of an enlightened policy in this regard would do something 'to mitigate for the elderly the various adverse social consequences of population mobility, and by making a major contribution to their welfare might well prove as economic as the building of old people's homes or units of sheltered housing'.[7]

CONCLUSIONS

Although the principal feature of the demography of the elderly in the coming 30 years is one of steady increase, particularly in the most dependent section of the population, i.e. the oldest, there are a number of demographic features that point to a better prospect for these elderly people. Some of the most important of these features are, perhaps luckily, inevitable, while some are susceptible to manipulation to the advantage of the elderly.

REFERENCES

1. Grundy E. (1987) This volume, p. 53.
2. Irvine R. E. (1987) This volume, p. 165.
3. Office of Population Censuses and Surveys (1983) *Census 1981*. London, HMSO.
4. Donaldson L. J., Clarke M. and Palmer R. L. (1983) *Health Trends* **15**, 58.

5. Carstairs V. and Morrison M. (1971) *Scottish Health Service Studies No. 19*. Edinburgh, Scottish Home and Health Department, Table 5.10.
6. Office of Population Censuses and Surveys (1981) *Population Projections 1978–2018*. PP2 No. 10. London, HMSO, Table 7b.
7. Roberston C., Gilmore A. J. J. and Caird F. I. (1975) *Health Bull.* **33**, 1.
8. Office of Population Censuses and Surveys (1985) *Population Projections 1983–2023*. PP2 No. 13. London, HMSO, Appdx Table 3 A1.

5. FUTURE PATTERNS OF MORBIDITY IN OLD AGE

Emily Grundy

INTRODUCTION

The concept of morbidity is an elusive one and the possible implications of a particular disease process for an individual or a population vary widely. Partly for this reason data on morbidity are difficult to collect and interpret; predicting future morbidity patterns poses even greater problems. Traditionally mortality data have been used as an indicator of the health of a population and theories about morbidity are closely related to the interpretation of mortality statistics. Although some have questioned the use of mortality data to make inferences about morbidity, particularly morbidity from chronic diseases,[1] it is useful to start any discussion of morbidity with a review of mortality trends, especially as past changes in vital rates have been so important in shaping the age structure of today's population, and morbidity, particularly from chronic conditions, is strongly age-related. Theories about the relationship between mortality and morbidity and about the process of ageing itself are also based on interpretations of trends in mortality.

The current older age structure of Britain and other developed countries is a result of the long-term fall in fertility, which formed part of the demographic transition from relatively high to low vital rates in the late nineteenth and early twentieth centuries.[2] Mortality rates fell substantially during this period, largely as a result of reductions in the death rate from infectious diseases; this involved the emergence of cardiovascular and cerebrovascular diseases and malignant neoplasms as the leading causes of death. The shift in the cause structure of death, sometimes described as the epidemiological transition, produced what Omran termed the 'age of degenerative and manmade diseases'.[3]

Figure 5.1, adapted from Preston's work,[4] shows the typical cause of death structure of mortality in populations whose average life expectancy at birth is 45 for males and 50 for females, as was the case in England and Wales at the beginning of the century, compared with populations with life expectancies at birth of 70 and 75, close to current levels of life expectancy at birth in this country. Some of the differences in the cause of death structure reflect improvements in diagnostic and coding procedures in low mortality populations and a corresponding reduction in deaths assigned to 'other and unknown' causes, but the overall picture is clear; in low mortality countries deaths from chronic diseases predominate while in populations with higher levels of mortality infectious diseases are far more important.

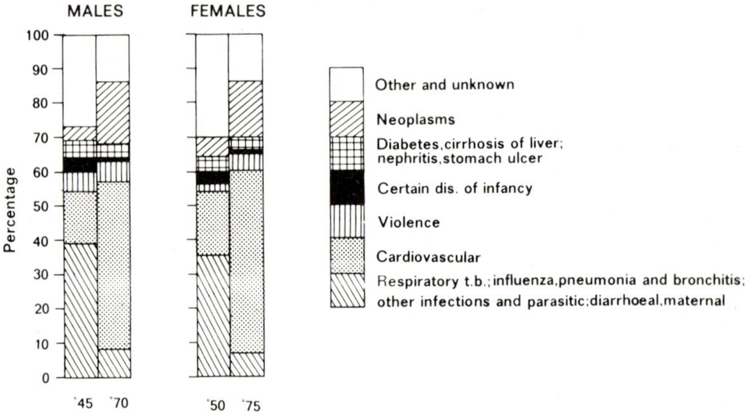

Fig. 5.1. Distribution of deaths by cause in populations with male expectations of life at birth of 45 and 70 years and female expectations of life at birth of 50 and 75 years.
Source: Adapted from Preston S. H. (1976) *Mortality Patterns in National Populations*. New York, Academic Press.

These historic changes in mortality affected age- and sex-groups differently. The largest proportionate falls in mortality were among the young, particularly infants and children, and, for reasons that are still not fully understood, the sex differential in mortality has increased as age-specific death rates have fallen.

These past falls in mortality are not the chief reason for today's older age structure, but recent changes in death rates at older ages have influenced the size and structure of the elderly population itself.[5] Historic falls in mortality at young ages are also one reason for the increase in the absolute, as opposed to the relative, number of old people in the past half-century. At present the age-groups over 80 are growing faster than any other; these groups comprise the survivors of the large Edwardian birth cohorts who were the first generations ever to have a greater than 50 per cent chance of reaching their 65th birthday.

THE INTERPRETATION OF TRENDS IN MORTALITY

Until relatively recently it was thought that once major improvements in nutrition, sanitation and housing had brought about substantial falls in infectious disease mortality, then further major improvements in life expectancy were unlikely.[3] Even recent population projections in some developed countries have been based entirely on anticipated trends in fertility and migration and have ignored the possibility of changes in death rates.[6] The view that further mortality falls were unlikely was held on the one hand by those who considered that 'endogenous' mortality rates from chronic diseases were inextricably associated with urbanization and industrial development and so largely irreducible through medical or environmental intervention,[7] and on the other by workers who believed that a biological limit to mortality reduction existed and had been more or less reached.[8] Even if diseases such as cancer were completely eradicated, the gain in life expectancy could be slight as those 'saved' from death from one particular cause were of an age where they would soon succumb to another unless a solution could be found to the problem of the 'deterioration and senescence of the cells of the human body'.[9] Further investigation of past and current trends in mortality has led to a revision of these views.

First of all it is now clear that although specific medical and technical interventions were not the chief cause of the nineteenth-century mortality transition, modern technologies and therapies can sometimes effect falls in death rates in the absence of major improvements in living standards. In some less developed countries innovations such as insect control have produced large reductions in death rates.[10] In the developed world, too, the introduction of sulphonamides, antibiotics and the spread of vaccination programmes contributed to substantial falls in mortality between 1930 and 1960.[11] More recently the fall in mortality from cardiovascular diseases in middle age, which started in the 1960s, particularly in the United States and Australia,[12] and the recent drop in the mortality of the elderly, have further invalidated the view that mortality rates had reached the lowest possible level.

The persistence of mortality differentials within and between developed countries also suggests that further improvements are possible. *Table* 5.1 shows that an 80-year-old man living in Sweden in the late 1970s would on average have a remaining life-span some 20 per cent longer than his counterpart in Scotland, while a 60-year old Canadian woman could expect to live 2 years longer than a woman from England or Wales.

Recent trends in mortality have thus led to a revision of previous ideas about an inevitable, socially induced limit to mortality decline and have also caused those who support the idea of a biological limit to the life-span to revise upwards estimates of what this limit might be.[13] This reinterpretation of past trends has not, however, produced a new consensus about the likely course of future mortality trends. Furthermore, some have argued that the relationship between mortality and morbidity is changing and that the policy emphasis should now focus on the reduction of chronic disease morbidity rather than on further reductions in death rates.

Table 5.1. Expectation of life at ages 60 and 80 in selected developed countries, 1975–1978

Country	*Expectation of life at age*			
	60 years		*80 years*	
	Male	*Female*	*Male*	*Female*
Canada	18·7	22·3	6·9	8·7
Denmark	17·3	21·6	6·4	7·9
England and Wales	15·8	20·4	5·6	7·1
Germany (West)	15·9	20·1	5·6	6·7
Hungary	15·1	18·5	5·1	6·0
Japan	18·0	21·5	6·2	7·4
Portugal	15·6	19·1	4·6	5·6
Scotland	14·9	19·5	5·3	7·0
Sweden	17·8	22·0	6·3	7·9
USA	17·1	22·0	7·0	9·2

Source: World Health Organization.

VIEWS ON TRENDS IN MORBIDITY

The most optimistic view of future morbidity trends is that put forward by Fries[14] and rests on the concept of a fixed biological limit to the life-span. The chief difference between Fries and earlier proponents of this view lies in the very precise predictions Fries makes about mortality change and the inferences he draws about morbidity. Fries argued that the limit to the life-span was about 115 and that in any population average life expectancy was unlikely to exceed 85. Future improvements in health, brought about by lifestyle changes and the acceptance of personal responsibility for health, would result not in further mortality decline but in a 'compression of morbidity' at the end of the life-span. Those who adopted the appropriate responsible attitude could hope to enjoy a vigorous life followed by a short period of ill health and then a 'natural death' resulting from biological senescence rather than a specific disease process.

The methodological, theoretical and empirical weaknesses in Fries' argument have been extensively commented on elsewhere and are not rehearsed here.[15–17] Suffice it to say that even if he is right about a fixed biological limit to the life-span, it is clear that no population is anywhere near the stage where it operates in the way he has suggested. Longitudinal studies of elderly people in developed societies have shown that the best predictors of mortality are the markers of established disease[18] or degree of functional capacity;[19] it has also been demonstrated that the period of pre-death morbidity is longest in those dying at older ages[20] and that the subgroups of populations with the highest mortality rates suffer the longest periods of disability.[21] Furthermore, far from reaching a mortality 'ceiling' many developed countries are experiencing continuing falls in death rates at advanced ages.[22,23]

Gruenberg and others[24,25] have put forward a view of future mortality and morbidity trends diametrically opposed to that of Fries. They argue that reductions in mortality at older ages are currently being achieved not by reducing the incidence of degenerative chronic diseases or retarding their progression, but by medical interventions that postpone the lethal sequelae of chronic diseases, such as pneumonia. These trends, it is argued, have had the effect of increasing the prevalence of chronic disease morbidity by lengthening the duration of ill-health episodes before death. Kramer warned that these developments could result in a 'pandemic of mental illness'.[25] Recent studies that have shown an increase in the survival of old people with dementia[26,27] and a rise in the prevalence of this condition in the population as a result of longer durations of the disease have lent support to this argument.[28]

Although the views of Fries on the one hand and Gruenberg on the other seem at variance, Manton[29] has pointed out that both share the opinion that the relationship between mortality and morbidity is changing and that the emphasis of public health initiatives should be on reducing chronic disease morbidity rather than mortality. Manton used United States multi-cause coded death registration data to examine variations in the frequency with which certain chronic diseases were mentioned at all compared with the frequency with which they featured as the underlying cause of death—in effect, a kind of chronic disease case fatality rate. This analysis led him to conclude that the prevalence of chronic diseases was increasing, but not as a result of the postponement of lethal sequelae. Rather, he suggested, the rate of progression of certain degenerative chronic diseases had slowed down, partly as a result of innovations such as hypertension control. People with chronic degenerative diseases were surviving to older ages and then dying of other causes with the initial chronic disease operating in only a contributory role.

The issues raised by these differing interpretations of current trends in mortality are complex and so it is appropriate to examine recent changes in mortality rates among the elderly.

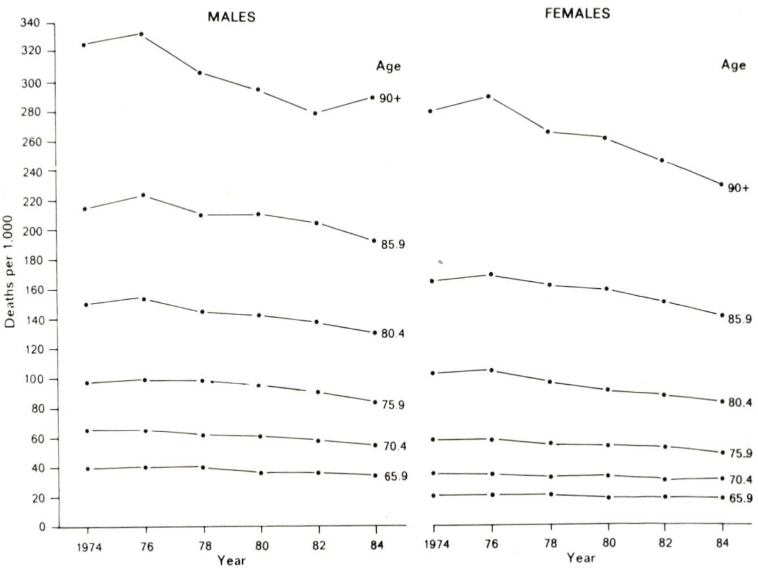

Fig. 5.2. Changes in mortality rates among the elderly in England and Wales, 1974–1984.

Figure 5.2 shows recent trends in mortality rates at older ages in England and Wales. Declines in mortality among the very old in what is a relatively short period have been considerable and show little sign of diminishing. If this drop in the death rate were the result of a narrowing in differentials in mortality at older ages as higher mortality groups 'caught up' with lower mortality groups, then this might suggest that the mortality of the most advantaged groups had fallen to an irreducibly low level. However, this does not seem to be the case; in the United States, for example, recent falls in death rates have been greatest among white females, leading to a widening rather than a narrowing of differentials. Socioeconomic differences in the chance of dying have also been shown to persist beyond the age of 65,[30] which itself suggests a continuing link between mortality and morbidity at older ages.

TRENDS IN MORBIDITY AT OLDER AGES IN BRITAIN

The chief national data on morbidity in Britain come from statistics on deaths and discharges from hospitals and admissions to psychiatric hospitals, from the surveys of consultations with general practitioners and from the health questions included in the General Household Survey (GHS). Hospital data relate to admissions or discharges rather than individual patients and so are of limited use in studying chronic disease morbidity because of the common pattern of multiple admissions. The decision to admit to or discharge from hospital also depends on a variety of social and environmental factors, as well as the availability of beds, which are not directly related to the severity of the disease. The surveys of general practice, while useful, relate to only two points in time and are based on information collected from general practices that may be atypical. This leaves the GHS as probably the best source of national data on trends in morbidity.

Since its inception in 1971 the GHS has included questions on longstanding illness, 'limiting' longstanding illness and illness causing short-term restricted activity. These indicators of morbidity are derived from answers to questions from an interviewer rather than from physical examination and, except in 1971, questions about specific diseases were not included.

Figure 5.3 shows trends in the proportion of people aged 65–74 and 75 and over who reported that they had a longstanding illness, a limiting longstanding illness or an illness that had restricted their activity in the 14 days prior to interview. Data for 1971, 1977 and 1978 are not shown as in these years the health questions were put differently; data on limiting longstanding illness are not available for 1972. The general trend in all of these rates has been upward, particularly among women aged 65–74. In 1983 63 per cent of this group reported that they had a longstanding illness compared with 48 per cent of those interviewed in 1972.[31] These increases appear alarming but there may be reasons other than changes in underlying morbidity that have influenced responses in the GHS. The increase in the proportion reporting longstanding illness might reflect changing expectations of health and a greater tendency to seek medical diagnosis and treatment for problems previously shrugged off as the inevitable consequence of ageing. A condition that has been acknowledged and named by a doctor is probably more likely to be remembered and reported in a survey than an undiagnosed illness. The GHS data on consultations with general practitioners do not show a consistent upward trend, although there is a suggestion of a rise in the proportion of elderly people attending outpatient departments, but general practitioners in 1983 may have been more likely to diagnose and treat illness in the elderly than they were a decade earlier. It is less obvious that these factors would affect the proportions reporting restricted activity in the 14 days prior to interview, but possibly increases in health awareness and in the kinds of activities normally carried out might have affected the response to this question in the GHS.

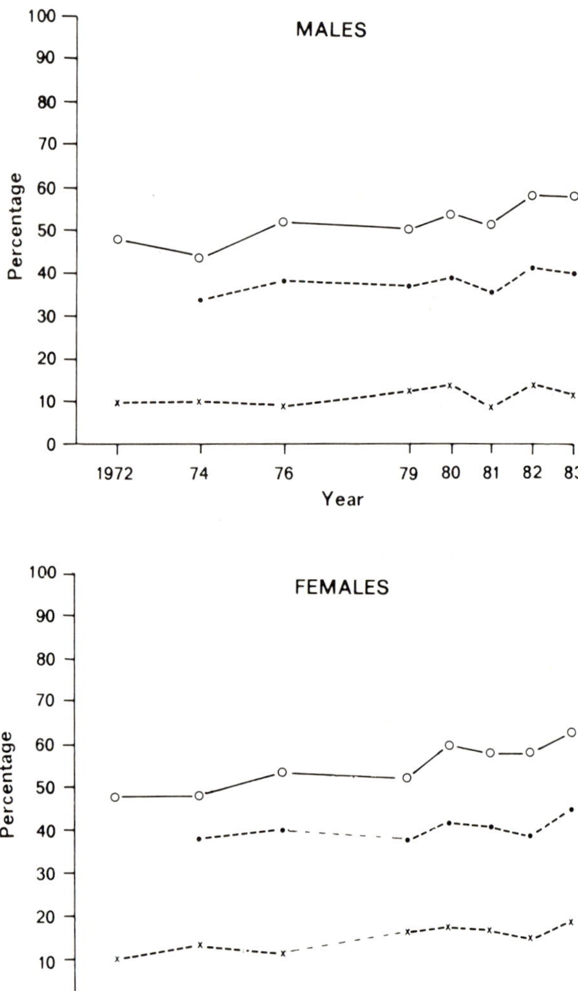

a

Fig. 5.3. Reported longstanding illness, limiting longstanding illness and restricted activity among 65–74-year-olds (*a*) and over-75s (*b*) in Britain, 1972–1983. *Source*: Office of Population Censuses and Surveys, *General Household Survey 1972–1983*. London, HMSO.

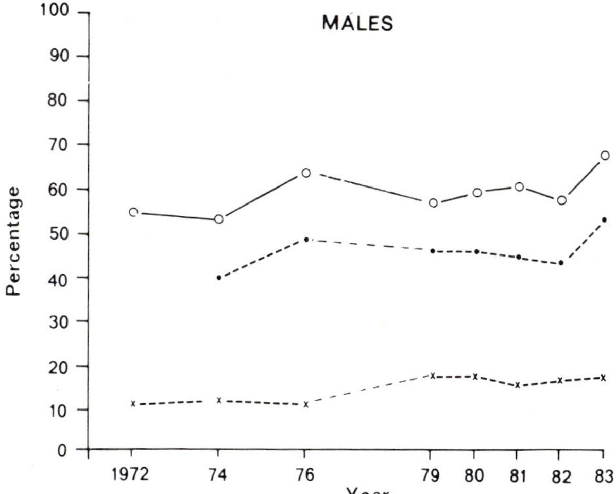

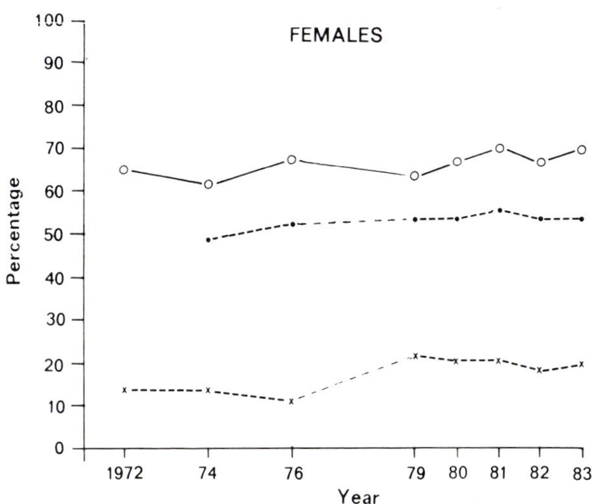

o—o Longstanding illness
•----• Limiting longstanding illness
x---x Restricted activity in preceding 14 days

b

The increases in reported longstanding illness among the elderly between 1972 and 1983 were in both absolute and relative terms less marked than increases in other age-groups, as shown in *Table* 5.2. Relative increases in the prevalence of chronic illness have been particularly marked among children. Increases in acute illness, as measured by restricted activity in the 14 days prior to interview, were also greater among children than among the elderly. Trends in morbidity in the United States, as measured in the United States National Health Interview Survey (NHIS), show a similar pattern. Colvez and Blanchet[32] analysed data from this survey for the period 1966–1976 and reported an increase in reported disability and short-term restricted activity among the under-65s but not among the elderly.

The increases in the reported prevalence of illness in the GHS may be a warning of real changes in morbidity, rather than a reflection of changing health standards, but if so it does not seem that it can reflect solely an increased prevalence of chronic disease among the elderly resulting from the postponement of lethal sequelae. If this hypothesis were true we would expect rises in reported illness to be greatest in the oldest age-groups rather than in the youngest.

Table 5.2. Changes in the reported prevalence of longstanding illness and restricted activity (in the 14 days prior to interview) between 1972 and 1983

Age	*Longstanding illness*				*Restricted activity*			
	Change in % reporting		*1983 rate as % of 1972 rate*		*Change in % reporting*		*1983 rate as % of 1972 rate*	
	Male	*Female*	*Male*	*Female*	*Male*	*Female*	*Male*	*Female*
0–4	+ 6	+ 6	220	300	+10	+8	300	233
5–15	+ 8	+ 7	189	217	+ 6	+6	200	220
16–44	+ 9	+10	164	177	+ 1	+5	114	163
45–64	+15	+14	152	145	+ 2	+6	122	167
65–74	+10	+15	121	131	+ 2	+9	120	190
75+	+13	+ 5	124	108	+ 7	+6	170	143
All ages	+11	+12	155	157	+ 4	+6	157	175

Source: Office of Population Censuses and Surveys (1974, 1985) *General Household Survey 1972* and *1983*. London, HMSO.

DIFFERENTIALS IN MORBIDITY

The GHS data can also be used to look at socioeconomic variations in reported morbidity. *Figure* 5.4 shows differences in longstanding illness, limiting longstanding illness and restricted activity by socioeconomic group among those aged 65 and over. The measure of socioeconomic group was based on current or last occupation or, for ever-married women, occupation of husband. Among men those in the

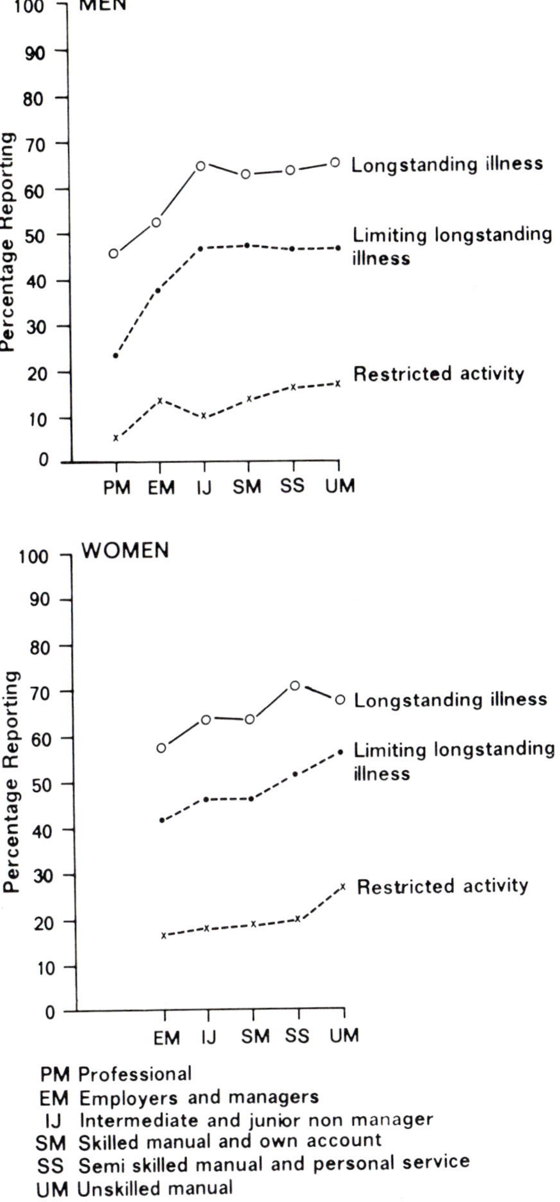

Fig. 5.4. Reported limiting longstanding illness and restricted activity among the population aged 65 and over by socioeconomic group in Britain, 1983.
Source: Office of Population Censuses and Surveys (1985) *General Household Survey 1983*. London, HMSO.

Table 5.3. Prevalence (%) of functional disability among elderly people in private households in Britain, 1980, and the proportion of elderly people resident in institutions in Britain, 1981

	Age (years)											
	65–69			*70–74*			*75–79*			*80+*		
	Male	*Female*	*Persons*	*Male*	*Female*	*Persons*	*Male*	*Female*	*Persons*	*Male*	*Female*	*Persons*
Functional disability												
Slight	18	26	22	24	28	26	31	34	33	24	25	24
Moderate	7	12	10	11	19	16	19	28	25	24	34	31
Severe	3	4	3	5	6	6	6	8	7	17	25	22
Resident in institution	1	1	1	2	2	2	3	4	4	8	14	12
Total with moderate/severe disability*	11	17	14	18	27	24	28	40	36	49	73	65

* Including residents in institutions.

Source: 1981 Census and Evandrou M., Arber S., Dale A. et al. (in press) In: Phillipson C., Bernard H. and Strang P. (eds) *Dependency and Interdependency in Old Age*. Beckenham, Croom Helm.

professional or employer and manager groups had markedly lower rates of longstanding illness and limiting longstanding illness than other groups. Social class gradients in all three measures of morbidity are also apparent among women. It is unlikely that these differences are the artificial result of variation in the reporting of illness, as one would expect those in the higher social groups to be more informed about health problems and so more, rather than less, likely to report ill health. There are of course other problems involved in interpreting these data connected with differences in the probability of surviving to age 65 and beyond, changes in the occupational structure that mean more recent cohorts include fewer manual workers and possibly also health-related occupational shifts in the pre-retirement period (although these would have less effect on the results shown for women). Despite these caveats it seems clear that reported morbidity among the over-65s, like mortality,[30] varies with socioeconomic status. In short, within sex-groups the risk of ill health and the risk of death among the elderly are positively associated with each other. Women however, have both lower mortality and higher morbidity rates than men.

MORBIDITY AND FUNCTIONAL DISABILITY

In 1980 the GHS had an expanded section on the elderly with questions on the ability to perform certain personal care and household activities.[33] These included eating, bathing, walking inside and outside, climbing stairs and cutting toenails. The proportions reporting an inability to carry out these tasks or that they needed help with them or could manage alone only with difficulty are very similar to the results of Hunt's survey[34] of the elderly at home carried out 4 years earlier. The answers to these questions in the GHS were used by Evandrou et al.[35] to derive an index of functional capacity based on the index used in Townsend and Wedderburn's 1962 study.[36] Evandrou et al. found that 8 per cent of all elderly people could be considered severely disabled, defined as being unable to manage or needing help with at least two out of six personal care or mobility functions and having difficulty with at least four. Forty-nine per cent of the sample had no disability in that they were able to carry out all six tasks without difficulty.

There were of course strong age variations in functional capacity; 25 per cent of women and 17 per cent of men aged 80 or over were classified as severely disabled compared with only 3 and 4 per cent of those aged 65–69. Conversely 34 and 17 per cent of men and women of 80 and over had no disability compared with 72 per cent and 59 per cent of the 65–69 age group.

The age-specific prevalence rates of slight, moderate and severe disability reported in Evandrou et al.'s study are shown in *Table* 5.3 together with the proportions recorded as resident in institutions in the 1981 Census. Visitors to institutions (including short-stay patients in hospitals) and resident staff have been excluded. Given the high rates of functional disability found in surveys of residents in old people's homes and hospitals,[37] it seems reasonable to assume that all of these old people living in institutions were at least moderately, if not severely, functionally disabled.

The high prevalence of severe or moderate functional disability among those aged 80 or over has serious implications for the future as the size of this age-group is projected to increase substantially. Twelve per cent of those aged 80 or over (and 19 per cent of those over 85) lived in institutions in 1981 and the 1980 GHS data anlaysed by Evandrou et al. show 53 per cent of the over-80s to be moderately or severely disabled.

However, there are some indications that the mobility and functional ability of the elderly living at home may have improved slightly. In the Townsend and Wedderburn survey,[36] which had an age composition very similar to that of the 1980 GHS, 9·1 per cent of respondents were categorized as severely disabled or bedfast (the definition of bedfast used implied less functional ability than those described as severely disabled) compared with 7·7 per cent of the 1980 sample. Townsend and Wedderburn also reported that 20 per cent of their sample were unable to go outside unaided compared with 15 per cent of respondents in Hunt's 1976 study of the elderly at home in England and Wales.[34] Variations in the proportion of the population in institutions cannot account for these differences as Census results show that in 1961 5 per cent of the over-65s in Britain permanently resided in institutions compared with 4 per cent in 1981.

Given the advances not just in geriatric and general medicine in the past 20 years but also in living standards among the elderly, it would be very disappointing if such a fall, however slight, had not occurred. This is particularly true as functional capacity depends to a considerable extent on the interaction between the individual and his or her environment. If an old person who lives in a centrally heated, purpose-built flat on one level says that he or she can only get around indoors with difficulty this implies a higher level of underlying morbidity and disability than would a similar response from an old person living in a poorly heated prewar dwelling with many steps and few amenities. Although housing standards among the elderly are still poor compared to those among the population as a whole, substantial improvements were made in the 1960s and 1970s. Only 20 per cent of households consisting of one person aged 60 or over had central heating in 1971; by 1983 this proportion was 54 per cent (the figures for all types of household are respectively 34 and 64 per cent).[31,38]

SOCIAL NETWORKS AND MORBIDITY

Health, as defined by the World Health Organization, includes social well-being. Apart from this being desirable in itself, a number of studies have shown that an individual's social circumstances influence physical and psychological health, as well as affecting the need for support from services. Berkman and Syme[39] investigated the relationship between social networks and mortality in a 9-year follow-up study of a sample of adults interviewed in Alameda County, California, in 1965. They constructed a social network index based on marital status, contacts with friends and relatives, church membership, and informal or formal association with a social group. Among women aged 60–69 at the start of the follow-up period the relative risk of dying for the most socially isolated compared to those with the most connections was 3; among men of the same age it was 1·8. Analyses based on the whole sample, which included younger respondents, showed that the associations between social networks and mortality were independent of self-reported physical health in the initial survey, year of death, socioeconomic status and health-related behaviour such as smoking, drinking, physical activity and use of preventive health services. Welin et al.[40] report similar findings from a 9-year follow-up study of Swedish men aged 50 or 60 at the start of the follow-up period. Household size was one of the variables independently related to mortality, with those in the largest households having the smallest mortality risk.

Little is known of the effect of social networks on the health of the oldest old and the problems involved in trying to identify such a relationship are greater as those with poor health will be more likely to move into larger households with relatives or into an institution. However, it seems safe to assume that emotional and social ties are just as important for the happiness of the oldest old as for those in their sixties and early seventies, and certainly the need for practical help from friends and relatives increases with age.

The proportion of old people living alone, and therefore perhaps at the greatest risk of social isolation, has increased substantially in the past 20 years. In 1962 30 per cent of women aged 65 or over lived alone compared with 45 per cent in 1980–1981.[41] This change is partly a result of the 'ageing' of the elderly population itself with a consequent increase in the proportion of widows and widowers. However, there have also been other changes in the residential patterns of elderly people and a large increase in the proportion of older people who head their own households rather than living in the households of others. In 1962 37 per cent of men and 45 per cent of women who were not currently married lived alone; by 1980–1981 these proportions had risen to respectively 65 and 72 per cent.[41] These changes do not reflect an 'abandonment' of the elderly by their relatives. The largest recent rises in household headship rates among the elderly occurred at a time when living standards among pensioners were rising and it seems likely that much of the increase in the proportion of old people living alone reflects a preference for residential independence wherever possible.

Future generations of elderly people will have an advantage over the current cohorts of very old people in that a smaller proportion will be childless. This is because of past increases in the propensity to marry and have children, which occurred after about 1940. Timaeus,[42] in a useful series of projections of the family and household status of the elderly, has estimated that while one-quarter of those women who reached their sixtieth birthday during 1971–1976 will have no living children by the time they die, this proportion will fall to 16 per cent among the cohort reaching 60 in the first half of the 1990s.

FUTURE TRENDS IN MORBIDITY

Three alternative views of current trends in morbidity were reviewed earlier in this paper. Of these three it seems safe to reject Fries' hypothesis of an imminent and dramatic fall in morbidity as there is no empirical evidence to support his view that lifestyle changes will lead to better health but have no effect on mortality. This leaves us with Gruenberg's pessimistic view that falls in mortality have been effected by medical interventions that have led to a postponement of the lethal sequelae of chronic diseases or Manton's more optimistic suggestion that the rate of progression of certain chronic diseases has decreased. The difference between these views is that, while both anticipate a rise in the age-specific prevalence of chronic disease morbidity, the former argument also suggests an increase in the severity of chronic disease (because of longer survival of the most seriously impaired) while the latter posits a reduction in the severity of chronic disease.

The data from the GHS and other sources reviewed here would tend to support the Manton hypothesis. The social groups with the highest mortality also report higher levels of morbidity, evidence pointing to a continuing association between morbidity levels and mortality in old age. The GHS data also show an increase in the prevalence of chronic disease, although this may partly reflect changing health expectations, while there is some evidence to suggest that rates of severe functional disability may have fallen slightly. Improvements in living standards and in therapeutic interventions aimed at promoting and enhancing functional ability or slowing the rate of progression of chronic disease may have made it easier for old people to preserve functional ability even when suffering from chronic disease. An old lady who has a hip replacement, for example, may still suffer from osteoarthritis but her functional capacity will be greatly improved.

Morbidity and mortality are both strongly age related and the next 20 years will see an increase in the prevalence of chronic diseases simply as a result of the increase in the number of very old people. Of particular concern will be future trends in dementia of the Alzheimer type. Dementia is very closely related to age and affects approximately 20 per cent of the over-80s,[43] the fastest growing age-group in the population. It is also the condition that above all others is likely to lead to institutionalization and the need for substantial support. Unfortunately there currently seems to be little hope of preventing dementia altogether, although an encouraging report from the Lundby study suggests that the incidence of older-onset dementia fell slightly between 1947–1957 and 1957–1972, possibly reflecting better nutrition and reduced exposure to infections among the later cohort.[44] Cohort differences are likely to be very important in many other respects as well. It may be that future generations reach old age in a healthier state and are less prone to chronic disease than current generations. On the other hand the health of the very old today may reflect their status as 'survivors'. Thus in the United States mortality rates among black people are lower than among the white population after the age of 75, and it is thought that this reflects selection effects that mean that only a particularly healthy subgroup of the black population attain old age.[45] As yet it seems quite impossible to predict what effect these cohort differences may have on the future health status of the elderly.

Table 5.4 shows two alternative projections of chronic disease morbidity and moderate or severe functional disability. All are based on the Office of Population Censuses and Surveys (OPCS) population projections that assume a 25 per cent fall in mortality among the elderly between 1983 and 2023.[46] The optimistic projection assumes that, despite the older age structure of the population aged 75 and over and past increases in reported longstanding morbidity, the 1983 levels of chronic disease for the age-groups 65–74 and 75+ will remain constant and the age-specific rates of moderate and severe functional disability shown in *Table* 5.3 will fall by 10 per cent by 2001 in the age-group 65–79 and by 5 per cent among the over-80s, as a result of advances in secondary prevention. The conservative projection assumes a 5 per cent increase in moderate and severe functional disability in the 80+ age-group and a 10 per cent increase in longstanding illness in the 75+ age-group, both increases reflecting the future older age composition of these groups.

To meet the assumptions made in the optimistic projection would involve real advances in the primary and secondary prevention of chronic disease and disability and the delivery of medical and other services. Even if these conditions were met there would be, in 1996, 305 000 more elderly people with chronic diseases than in 1983 and an additional 98 000 who were moderately or severely functionally impaired. The more conservative projection implies an increase of over 500 000 in the number of elderly people with longstanding illnesses by the beginning of the next century and over 380 000 more old people with moderate or severe functional disabilities.

Table 5.4. Projected numbers of elderly people (65+) with longstanding illness and moderate or severe functional disability, 1983–2001

Projection type and morbidity indicator	*1983*	*1986*	*Year* *1991*	*1996*	*2001*
Optimistic					
Longstanding illness					
N (000s)	5282	5450	5593	5587	5514
% change	100	103	106	106	104
% of population aged 65+	64	64	64	64	65
Moderate/severe functional disability					
N (000s)	2607	2683	2730	2700	2626
% change	100	103	105	104	101
% of population aged 65+	32	32	31	31	31
Conservative					
Longstanding illness					
N (000s)	5282	5492	5710	5780	5789
% change	100	104	108	109	110
% of population aged 65+	64	65	66	67	68
Moderate/severe functional disability					
N (000s)	2607	2738	2887	2960	2991
% change	100	105	110	114	115
% of population aged 65+	32	32	33	34	35

Source: Office of Population Censuses and Surveys (1985) *Population Projections 1983–2023*. London, HMSO.

CONCLUSION

The ageing of Britain's population has profound implications for the development, delivery and financing of health and welfare services. In 1983, for example, National Health Service expenditure per caput for those aged 75 and over was more than four times per caput expenditure for the population as a whole.[47] Trends in reported morbidity and mortality suggest a continuing strong link between the two and continuing scope for improvements in the health of currently disadvantaged groups of elderly people. Although a rise in morbidity from chronic diseases seems inevitable and it is probably unrealistic to hope that chronic diseases in later life can be prevented altogether, much can be done to preserve functional ability in the old and to promote autonomy even among the very disabled.[48] If this is to achieved, however, much will also have to be done in the fields of basic and applied research and service development. There is also an urgent need to expand and improve domiciliary and residential health and welfare services to meet the needs of the growing population of severely disabled old people.

REFERENCES

1. Beeson P. B. (1977) *Milbank Mem. Fund Q.* **55**, 365.
2. Grundy E. (1983) *J. Am. Geriatr. Soc.* **31**, 325.
3. Omran A. R. (1971) *Milbank Mem. Fund Q.* **49**, 509.
4. Preston S. H. (1976) *Mortality Patterns in National Populations.* New York, Academic Press.
5. Benjamin B. and Overton E. (1981) *Popul. Trends* **23**, 22.
6. Australian Bureau of Statistics (1978) *Projections of the Population of Australia 1978 to 2011.* Canberra, Australian Bureau of Statistics.
7. Dubos R. (1965) *Man Adapting.* New Haven, Yale University Press.
8. Bourgeois-Pichat J. (1952) *Population* **7**, 381.
9. Keyfitz N. (1978) *Am. J. Public Health* **68**, 954.
10. Gray R. (1974) *Popul. Studies* **28**, 205.
11. Preston S. H. (1975) *Popul. Studies* **29**, 231.
12. Dwyer T. and Hetzel B. S. (1980) *Int. J. Epidemiol.* **9**, 65.
13. Bourgeois-Pichat J. (1978) *Popul. Bull. UN* **11**, 12.
14. Fries J. F. (1980) *N. Engl. J. Med.* **303**, 130.
15. Bromley D., Isaacs A. and Bytheway B. (1982) *Ageing Soc.* **2**, 283.
16. Grundy E. (1984) *Br. Med. J.* **288**, 663.
17. Schneider E. L. and Brody J. A. (1983) *N. Engl. J. Med.* **309**, 854.
18. Campbell J., Diep C., Reinken J. et al. (1985) *J. Epidemiol. Community Health* **39**, 337.
19. Warren D. and Knight R. (1982) *J. Epidemiol. Community Health* **36**, 220.
20. Isaacs B., Livingstone M. and Neville Y. (1971) *Lancet* **i**, 1115.
21. Wilkins R. and Adams O. (1983) *Am. J. Public Health* **73**, 1073.
22. Myers G. C. (1979) In: Donald J. M., Everitt A. V. and Wheeler P. J. (eds) *Ageing in Australia.* Sydney, Australian Association of Gerontology.
23. Rosenwaike I., Yaffe N. and Sagi P. C. (1980) *Am. J. Public Health* **70**, 1074.
24. Gruenberg E. M. (1977) *Milbank Mem. Fund Q.* **55**, 3.
25. Kramer M. (1980) *Acta Psychiatr. Scand.* **62**, Suppl. 285.
26. Blessed G. and Wilson I. D. (1982) *Br. J. Psychiatry* **141**, 59.
27. Christie A. B. (1982) *Br. J. Psychiatry* **140**, 154.
28. Gruenberg E. M. and Hagnell O. (1976) In: Levy I. (ed.) *Stress and Disease: Aging and Old Age.* Proceedings of the WHO Symposium Society, Stockholm, 1976.
29. Manton K. G. (1982) *Milbank Mem. Fund Q.* **60**, 183.

30. Fox A. J., Goldblatt P. O. and Jones D. R. (1985) *J. Epidemiol. Community Health* **39**, 1.
31. Office of Population Censuses and Surveys (1985) *The General Household Survey 1983*. London, HMSO.
32. Colvez A. and Blanchet M. (1981) *Am. J. Public Health* **71**, 464.
33. Office of Population Censuses and Surveys (1982) *The General Household Survey 1980*. London, HMSO.
34. Hunt A. (1978) *The Elderly at Home*. London, HMSO.
35. Evandrou M., Arber S., Dale A. et al. (1986) In: Phillipson C., Bernard H. and Strang P. (eds.) *Dependency and Interdependency in Old Age*. Beckenham, Croom Helm, p. 150.
36. Townsend P. and Wedderburn D. (1965) *The Aged in the Welfare State*. London, G. Bell and Sons.
37. Clarke M., Hughes A. O., Dodd K. J. et al. (1979) *Health Trends* **11**, 17.
38. Office of Population Censuses and Surveys (1973) *The General Household Survey 1971*. London, HMSO.
39. Berkman L. and Syme S. (1979) *Am. J. Epidemiol.* **109**, 186.
40. Welin L., Svardsudd K., Ander-Peciva S. et al. (1985) *Lancet* **i**, 915.
41. Wall R. (1984) *Ageing Soc.* **4**, 483.
42. Timaeus I. (1986) *Ageing Soc.* **6,** 271.
43. Kay D., Beamish P. and Roth M. (1964) *Br. J. Psychiatry* **110**, 146.
44. Hagnell O., Lanke J., Rorsman B. et al. (1981) *Neuropsychobiology* **7**, 201.
45. Manton K. and Stallard E. (1981) *Hum. Biol.* **53**, 47.
46. Office of Population Censuses and Surveys (1985) *Population Projections 1983–2023*. London, HMSO.
47. Central Statistical Office (1986) *Social Trends 1986*. London, HMSO.
48. Grimley Evans J. (1984) *J. Chron. Dis.* **37**, 353.

Part II

DERMATOLOGY OF OLD AGE

6. THE BIOLOGY OF AGEING SKIN

Andrew Y. Finlay

INTRODUCTION

The appearance of a person's skin is a very good guide to his or her age. This statement is obvious, but wrong. It is essential to understand the reasons why it is incorrect before attempting to grasp the concepts of skin ageing.

The statement seems to be correct because the areas of skin of which we are most aware socially are the face and hands. These sites are subject to the harshest effects of a lifetime's unprotected encounter with the environment. They are battered daily by ultraviolet radiation, swept by our polluted atmosphere and further insulted by our attempts at becoming clean or looking attractive. The havoc that these events play on our skin have an additive effect over the years, initially subtly, and later more grossly, altering our skin so that there is indeed an association between age and the appearance of the skin in these exposed sites.

Why then is the statement still wrong? To get to the bottom of this I would respectfully ask you to lower your trousers or skirt so exposing an expanse of protected, unsullied skin, of exactly the same age as the skin on your face. Here you will find the effects, if any, of ageing alone. The 'ageing' effects that we all recognize on the face are exposed as being fraudulent, an attempt by the environment to confuse us. Truly to understand the biology of ageing skin it is essential to try to separate true ageing from the cumulative effects of the environment. Both are of importance.

Apart from the confusion between environmentally induced changes and true ageing, other pitfalls for investigators include confusion between ageing changes and manifestations of age-associated diseases and confusion between ageing changes and age-associated hormonal changes.[1]

Although the changes seen in light-protected skin are less obvious, there are in fact many differences between even the protected skin of a 70-year-old and the skin of a child. Changes can be detected at all levels of the skin both in structure and function.

SUBCUTANEOUS TISSUE

The distribution of subcutaneous fat profoundly influences the appearance of skin. Lift up a 'pinch' of skin from a teenager's forearm and then do the same to a 70-year-old. The younger person's skin feels thick and well cushioned but the older skin seems flimsy, easily stretchable and thin. These differences are caused by a combination of changes in all levels of the skin but most obviously by the differences in the subcutaneous fat. Subcutaneous fat is considerably reduced in most sites with age. The functional significances of this change include a contribution to the reduced cold tolerance of the elderly and a reduced ability to withstand simple daily knocks because of the reduction in subcutaneous cushioning.

THE DERMIS

The dermis provides our personal inner leather lining; its physical properties are fundamental to the strength and flexibility of human skin. The major component of the dermis, collagen, is produced by fibroblasts and changes are seen in both fibroblasts and collagen in the elderly. Other important components of the dermis include elastin and blood vessels, and the dermis is of course the home of various adnexal structures. All show changes associated with ageing, several of which are of fundamental importance.

Collagen

The main component of the dermis is collagen. The structure of collagen itself alters with time after synthesis: the collagen cross-links are formed and the immediate product is stabilized. These relatively rapid processes are followed by a slow, modest increase in shrinkage temperature of the collagen and stabilization of the cross-links. These are changes associated with short-term collagen ageing at any stage of life and need to be distinguished from changes in the collagen specifically associated with very old age.[2] Human and animal studies indicate that after injury to the skin, there is slower contraction of open wounds in the elderly. Collagen remodelling occurs later in older animals. Despite these observations, in clinical practice operations can be performed safely on the elderly and any delay in wound healing is insignificant compared to the increased risk of other operative and postoperative complications in this age-group.[3]

Skin Thickness

The collagen content of dermis provides an important component of skin thickness and the reduction in collagen content contributes to the reduction of skin thickness with age.[4] However, the concept of 'skin thickness' is especially ambiguous, as the term is meaningless unless it is clearly defined which layers of the skin are being measured. Different techniques measure different parameters and clinically both very hyperkeratotic skin can be called 'thick', where the stratum corneum alone is affected, and sclerodermatous skin can be called 'thick', where the dermis is increased in depth.

A radiographic technique measuring dermal thickness showed that there is reduction in skin thickness in older age-groups of both sexes.[5] This has been confirmed using ultrasound, a technique that can also be used to measure dermal and epidermal thickness separately,[6] and a reduction of 20 per cent of skin thickness in males and 14 per cent in females was detected when the over-70 age-group was compared to young adults. This study also clearly demonstrated that females have lower skin thickness than males in all age-groups.

Dermal Fibroblasts

In vitro studies of skin fibroblast cultures are a useful model for the investigation of human cellular ageing. The ability of skin fibroblasts to replicate decreases as a function of the age of the donor, but some aspects of skin fibroblasts such as protein and RNA content are not affected by age. The response of cultured fibroblast cells to insulin-like hormones also decreases with age.[7] It remains an intriguing possibility that the ability of dermal fibroblasts to replicate well in culture may correlate with good wound healing.[8] A clinical parallel consequence of the reduced ability of fibroblasts to replicate with age is the slight retardation of the superficial wound healing in persons aged over 65 as mentioned earlier.[9]

Changes with ageing in dermal fibroblast function and collagen may therefore contribute to changes in strength and flexibility of skin. Fortunately these changes are not of significant clinical importance.

Dermal Elastin and Wrinkling

There is a dense network of elastin fibres throughout the dermis that contributes specifically to important physical properties of the skin such as extensibility and ability to return to normal contour after deformation. Dermal elastin alters with age, resulting in clinically visible changes. Even in sun-protected sites, the skin wrinkles easily and becomes thin with a decrease in subcutaneous fat as age increases. These wrinkles are not permanent but disappear easily when stretched. The elastic fibre network in skin begins to show structural deterioration from the age of 30, slowly increasing with time.[10]

In sun-protected sites in persons over the age of 50, the terminal elastic fibre arcades in the upper dermis become thicker, with large amounts of 8- to 11-nm diameter microfilaments.[11] In addition there is an increase in the complexity of shape and arrangements of the elastic fibres, including flattening and branching. There is also an increase in the roughness of the surface of the fibres and a decrease in the interfibre space.[12] Eventually the whole elastic fibre structure shrinks and sags, no longer supporting even the epidermis. These findings are much more accentuated and are seen much earlier in sun-exposed sites.[13]

Scanning electron microscopy reveals that the surface of the dermal elastic fibres consists of fibrils separated by furrows. In aged skin the fibrils become thinner and the interfibrillar material is increased.[14] The elastic fibres in fact become so thin that they may not be seen easily on light microscopy. These changes, which are seen in fine wrinkles, are also seen in all areas of ageing skin and are therefore not specific to the wrinkles.[15] Deterioration of the elastic tissue network results in the skin losing the ability to snap back into its original state after deformation, becoming looser and excessive.[16]

In sun-exposed skin there are major changes in the architecture of the papillary dermis, with elastic microfilaments being replaced by very large amounts of tightly packed collagen fibrils parallel to the skin surface. These changes are seen on light microscopy as a normal layer of collagen in the upper dermis, immediately beneath the epidermis, beneath which is abnormally staining collagen indicative of long-term sun damage. This upper layer, known as the 'Grenz zone', therefore shows changes similar to those seen in scar tissues, and so the Grenz zone may be a microscar.[11]

It is therefore well established that there are major changes with age in both elastin and collagen in the dermis. These changes are much more obvious in sun-exposed sites.

Receptor Organs in Dermis

Cutaneous nerve endings and receptor organs do not reach a stationary conditon after their initial development but retain the capacity for renewal. Meisner's corpuscles progressively become reduced in number and increased in length continuously from birth to old age but no evidence of true 'senescence' has been demonstrated in nerve endings or receptor organs.[17] Cutaneous nerves, eccrine sweat glands, axillary apocrine glands and lactiferous glands are not affected by age.

Sebaceous Glands

Of all the adnexal structures contained in the skin, perhaps the sebaceous gland shows the greatest variation with age. Physically small and functionally in first gear in infancy, adolescence brings a massive acceleration in size and output with gradual decline thereafter.

Usually there is a good correlation between the size of the sebaceous glands and the rate of sebum production, but on the face of the elderly less sebum is produced by large glands. The size of facial sebaceous glands increases with age although the activity of sebaceous glands in the elderly is lower than in young adults and surface lipid levels fall.[18]

The production of skin surface lipids by the sebaceous glands is under the direct influence of circulating androgenic steroids. During adolescence lipid production reaches a maximum by the age of 15. It has been suggested that skin surface lipids are produced at the same level until the age of 60 in males, after which time there is a progressive reduction; in women the fall-off in production is more gradual, starting at the age of 40 years and eventually reaching the same low level by the age of 80.[19] However, Jacobsen et al.[20] using a different technique to measure sebaceous wax ester secretion rates, demonstrate that the decline of sebaceous gland activity with age is a gradual process in both sexes with a more rapid decline in women (32 per cent per decade) than in men (23 per cent per decade). Eventually in the very elderly the skin surface lipid production is similar to that in children. The gradual reduction may be explained by a decline in sebaceous gland responsiveness to circulating androgens rather than by a decline in levels of circulating androgens.

The final outcome is that the production of skin surface lipids in the elderly adult is much less than in a younger person. This may contribute to changes in skin texture, and provides an argument for the use of emollients in the 'dry' skin of the elderly.

Blood Supply

An adequate blood supply to an organ is usually vital to its survival and the skin is no exception to this rule. Both vessel numbers and blood flow to the skin are reduced in the elderly. Luckily the skin is so well served by its complex vasculature that in most areas significant functional changes do not result, but at some sites, in particular the lower legs, local poor cutaneous blood flow certainly contributes to ulceration or makes healing more difficult.

Tests used to demonstrate reduced dermal blood supply in the elderly include dermal clearance studies of dyes such as sodium fluorescein or radio-labelled material. These tests are strictly measuring the functional ability of substances to be cleared from an area of skin by the blood supply and do not necessarily directly relate to rate of total blood flow through an area, as other features such as vascular permeability also contribute to changes in clearance. However, smaller blood vessels in aged skin are seen much less frequently on microscopy and elderly skin is often pale, observations supporting the view that cutaneous blood supply in the elderly is reduced. The dramatic reduction in superficial capillaries in the elderly is very striking, even in the sun-protected genital mucocutaneous areas, where there is collapse, disintegration and even total disappearance of vessels of the microcirculation.[13] In vulval skin no vessel obliteration was found and only very slight thickening of the vessel walls was seen after the age of 55.[21]

Veil cells are flat cells that surround all the dermal microvessels, totally external to the vessel wall. In a sample of aged buttock skin the veil cells were underdeveloped laterally so that they did not cover the vessel as well as normal veil cells.[22] This demonstrates another cellular anatomical change with age; the functional significance of this finding is not clear, but the decreased amount of normal membrane around aged vessels may be related to the number and degree of cytoplasmic development of the veil cells rather than to differences in veil cell metabolic activity.

DERMO-EPIDERMAL JUNCTION

The junction of dermis and epidermis is not just an anatomical division that allows dermatological medical artists free licence to draw wavy lines. It is in fact a three-dimensional interface with a variety of functions; its shape and integrity alter with age.

In a young person the dermo-epidermal junction is a three-dimensional relief of valleys, mountains and craters. There is a progressive flattening out of this bas-relief, which takes place much more quickly in sun-exposed areas. Scanning electron microscope studies show that with age there is a progressive change in the gross configuration of the dermo-epidermal interface with loss of dermal valleys and flattening and widening of dermal papillae. In the very elderly the junction is virtually completely flat at most sites. In young skin the basal epidermal cells have numerous basal microvilli, but these microvilli become severely reduced in the elderly.[13] An almost flat dermo-epidermal junction and excess amounts of lamina densa with attached anchoring fibrils are characteristic of both unexposed and exposed senile skin, suggesting that these alterations are the result of intrinsic ageing. The flat dermo-epidermal junction may contribute to the reduced ability of elderly skin to withstand lateral shearing forces, but the reduplication of the lamina densa–anchoring fibril complex may compensate in part for this by resulting in improved bonding.[11]

In vulval skin there is a gradual increase in the size and number of rete ridges until the seventh decade, followed by a regression to the pre-pubertal pattern.[21]

When the dermo-epidermal junction is viewed at a higher power, the basal lamina is seen at the interface between the dermis and epidermis. It has several functions including physical support for the epidermis and adhesion of the epidermis to the dermis.[23] The basal lamina may also influence epidermal differentiation and proliferation and provide a template for epidermal repair. The basal lamina may also alter with age and there is a loss of basal lamina corrugations. This correlates well with the decreased adherence of epidermis and dermis in senescent skin.

Surprisingly, therefore, although the gross changes seen in skin with age reflect primarily gross changes in the dermis, epidermis and subcutaneous fat, even a localized area such as the dermo-epidermal junction does exhibit significant ageing changes.

THE EPIDERMIS

The results of evolution never cease to amaze. The epidermis is a brilliant concept, overcoming at a single stroke two crucially important problems that would otherwise have prevented human beings from crawling around, as we do, in a hostile dry environment. First, the epidermis acts to produce the stratum corneum which, although very thick, is also very impermeable to water. Our body's internal watery environment is therefore protected and we can survive on land. Second, and equally crucially, the epidermis is constantly renewing the stratum corneum so defeating most ageing processes. The stratum corneum is the final frontier between ourselves and our surroundings and is therefore constantly traumatized. A plastic sheet in its place would rapidly become punctured and tattered; the process of renewal is essential.

Epidermal Cell Production

Methods of measuring epidermal cell production depend on techniques such as tritiated thymidine autoradiography; some controversy surrounds the interpretation of results obtained in these studies because of different views about the ratio of dividing and inactive basal cells. There is some scanty evidence to suggest that the rate of epidermal cell production decreases with age.[24] An increase of stratum corneum renewal time (14 days in young men and 26 in elderly men) in old age[25] is compatible with this. Epstein and Maibach,[26] however, found no change in epidermal cell renewal time with advancing age.

There are specific protective devices in the epidermis to cope with the constant onslaught of ultraviolet (UV) radiation in sun-exposed sites. Without constant surveillance of repair of UV-induced damage the skin would rapidly degenerate with the formation of multiple malignancies, as in xeroderma pigmentosum where DNA repair is abnormal.[27] In normal skin there are multiple pathways for the repair of the damaged human DNA of the crucially important dividing basal cells. In black skin where melanin provides major protection, these repair mechanisms are sufficient to result in a very low incidence of cutaneous malignancy even in the elderly. But in white skin, the repair mechanisms can be effectively overwhelmed and the incidence of malignancy is much greater.

In vitro studies of cultured epidermal keratinocytes from donors of different ages have shown no differences in the time course for repair of keratinocytes with damaged DNA after UV irradiation.[28] It had been suggested that a reduced capacity, with increasing age, of keratinocytes to recover by excision repair of DNA following UV damage may have contributed to an acceleration of ageing changes in the elderly; this seems unlikely, but it is not known whether other cellular recovery responses to damaged DNA are also unrelated to age.

Chronic sun exposure appears to accelerate ageing by several different mechanisms. It is known, for example, that the life-span of cultured keratinocytes is decreased by chronic sun exposure. UV exposure therefore accelerates ageing in human skin by this recognized *in vitro* criterion of ageing. Human fetal fibroblasts have a maximum life-span of approximately 50 generations,[29] and the effects of environmental influences may either alter the rate of division of cells or reduce the total number of potential generations.

In a study comparing sun-exposed (pre-auricular) and sun-protected (postauricular) skin, keratinocyte cultures from the sun-exposed sites had a shorter *in vitro* life-span, and focal abnormalities of keratinocyte proliferation and alignment were seen on electron microscopy, especially in the cultures from sun-exposed sites.[30]

Epidermal Histology

In unexposed skin, the epidermis becomes thinner with age but the fine structural features of the spinous and granular layers and corneocytes are similar to those seen in young people.[11] There are very few age-associated cytological changes detectable in the epidermis.

The epidermal Langerhans' cell population measured in sun-exposed sites is half that of sun-protected areas. Although Langerhans' cell numbers are known to decrease following exposure to UV light, the midwinter timing of this study demonstrated that suppression of Langerhans' cell density by repeated sun exposure may persist indefinitely.[30]

There are clear gradual changes with age in the basic histometric parameters of epidermis.[31] Mean keratinocyte height slowly becomes smaller with age and mean epidermal thickness (in cell numbers) becomes less at some sites. Corneocyte area tends to increase with age. These findings indicate that there is a continuous decrease in population size of the epidermis with increasing age and that epidermal cells also lose vertical height and 'volume'. The increase in surface area of corneocytes with increasing age possibly reflects an increased stratum corneum transit time with increased flattening of corneocytes.[32] In contrast it has been suggested that the vulval stratum corneum gradually becomes thicker with advancing age.[21]

DRY SKIN AND THE STRATUM CORNEUM

A sensation of 'dryness' of the skin is almost inevitable in people over the age of 70. The physical properties described loosely as 'dryness' are in fact a combination of properties that include flexibility, true water content and, most importantly, roughness of the surface. Good explanations for the increase in dryness sensation with age are lacking.

Attempts have been made to measure one aspect of what is perceived clinically as dryness, the water content of the stratum corneum. This is difficult enough *in vitro* but poses much greater problems *in vivo*. Kligman[9] has demonstrated that the ability of the stratum corneum to hold water increases with age and there is less transepidermal water loss in the elderly. Other investigators have described a technique that uses the effect that changes in water content have on the propagation and attenuation of low-frequency shear waves in skin. This method has been used to demonstrate that the stratum corneum and upper epidermis of aged skin have a lower water content than the skin of younger men.[33] This study measured the water content of the dorsum of the hand and so any changes detected may have been related also to sun exposure.

However, perhaps the most important aspect of understanding the concept of dry skin in the elderly is that dry skin does not necessarily have a low water content. Be aware that in the production of 'dryness' changes in water content of the stratum corneum are not as important as changes of surface roughness.

MECHANICAL PROPERTIES OF SKIN

It is obvious from the most superficial handling of skin of the young and the old that the mechanical properties of skin change with age. The ability of skin to withstand stretching and compression largely depends on the viscoelastic properties of the dermis and in particular on the elastic network and the geometry of the collagen. A variety of industrial testing methods have been applied to skin to define stress–

strain curves, compression creep curves and other aspects of the physical properties of skin. These tests can be carried out more easily *in vitro* with excised skin; *in vivo* testing is more difficult but reflects reality more accurately as the effects of the surrounding tissues that hold or deform skin locally are maintained during testing. There is a progressive loss with age in the elastic recovery of skin that can be explained by the degenerative changes in the dermal elastin network. There is also a progressive increase with age in the time required for viscoelastic recovery from great stresses. This ageing change may be due to changes in the collagen network and its immediate supporting environment.[34]

In the extremely elderly the changes in mechanical properties of the skin are seen most strikingly as the very slow recovery of skin that has only very mildly been stretched or deformed.

EXTERNAL AND SYSTEMIC INFLUENCES ON THE SKIN

There are a variety of different 'environmental' influences on the skin that potentially may have an additive effect and therefore exert age-related changes. The most obvious external influences are UV radiation and direct contact with a multitude of different substances, some of which are either irritant or potential allergens. Fortunately the constant renewal of the epidermis results in there being no obvious cumulative additive irritant effect over the years. However, in those people working in industry, there seems to be an increased susceptibility to minor irritants.[35] When formally tested, reactions to the irritants thymoquinone and crotonaldehyde are similar in all age-groups, but reactions to croton oil are less in the elderly,[36] and Grove et al.[37] demonstrated that older individuals tend to be less reactive to a variety of irritants.

'Systemic' influences may also be important as inappropriate diet and smoking may affect cutaneous vasculature and systemic disease and drugs may directly affect otherwise normal skin. This was illustrated in a recent quiz[38] in which 12 close-up photographs of mostly elderly faces were shown and the challenge was to identify which patients were smokers. It was simple to score high marks, confirming a clinical observation that the skin of heavy smokers shows subtle textural changes.

ASSESSMENT OF 'PHYSIOLOGICAL AGE'

Throughout history doctors, quacks and soothsayers have attempted to use the skin as a guide to other truths. The search is still on and methods are sought to use functional properties of the skin as a measure of 'physiological' ageing.

When the irritant ammonium hydroxide is applied to the skin the initial formation of microvesicles occurs more quickly in 60- to 75-year-olds than in young adults, but in contrast it takes much longer for full blisters to occur in the elderly age-group.[39] The increased rate of initial formation of microvesicles may be dependent on increased appendageal diffusion in the elderly, and the longer time taken for full blister formation may be partly caused by the decreased microvasculature in elderly skin.[9] In the study by Grove et al.[39] the subjects who failed to blister looked older than their age and the authors suggest that the blistering time technique may give information on the 'physiological' age of the skin.

Nail Growth

Linear nail growth rate decreases in humans by 50 per cent over a life-span of 75 years. There are periods of slow decline of nail growth rate alternating with periods of rapid decline with an approximately 7-year periodicity.[40] Nail growth rate itself can therefore only be used as a guide to physiological ageing if this periodicity is clearly understood.

CONCLUSION

Despite this alarming catalogue of changing and deteriorating skin anatomy and function, people rarely die from old skin. A host of complex functions persist much more successfully than in many other organs, despite the skin having to survive at the battle zone between the protected, warm, moist internal environment of the body and the cold outside world. Elderly skin deserves some congratulation.

FURTHER READING

For a more detailed and for the most authoritative account of the biology of ageing skin the reader is recommended to Dr Gilchrest's recent book,[1] the first of its kind to deal comprehensively with cutaneous gerontology.

REFERENCES

1. Gilchrest B. A. (1984) *Skin and Aging Processes*. Boca Raton, Florida, CRC Press.
2. Bentley J. P. (1969) *J. Invest. Dermatol.* **73**, 80.
3. Goodson W. H. and Hunt T. K. (1979) *J. Invest. Dermatol.* **73**, 88.
4. Black M. M., Bottoms E. and Shuster S. (1970) *Eur. J. Clin. Invest.* **1**, 127.
5. Black M. M. (1969) *Br. J. Dermatol.* **81**, 661.
6. Tan C. Y., Statham B., Marks R. et al. (1982) *Br. J. Dermatol.* **106**, 657.
7. Goldstein S. (1979) *J. Invest. Dermatol.* **73**, 19.

8. Schneider E. L. (1979) *J. Invest. Dermatol.* **73**, 15.
9. Kligman A. M. (1985) *J. Invest. Dermatol.* **113**, 37.
10. Braverman I. M. and Fonkerko E. (1982) *J. Invest. Dermatol.* **78**, 434.
11. Lavker R. M. (1979) *J. Invest. Dermatol.* **73**, 59.
12. Tsuji T. and Hamada T. (1981) *Br. J. Dermatol.* **105**, 57.
13. Montagna W. and Carlisle K. (1979) *J. Invest. Dermatol.* **73**, 47.
14. Tsuji T. (1985) *Clin. Exp. Dermatol.* **10**, 545.
15. Tsuji T., Yorifuji T., Hayashi Y. et al. (1986) *Br. J. Dermatol.* **114**, 329.
16. Kligman A. M., Zheng P. and Lavker R. M. (1985) *Br. J. Dermatol.* **113**, 37.
17. Cauna N. (1985) In: Montagna W. (ed.) *Advances in Biology of the Skin. Vol. 6, Ageing.* Oxford, Pergamon Press.
18. Plewig G. and Kligman A. M. (1978) *J. Invest. Dermatol.* **70**, 314.
19. Nazzaro-Porro M., Passi S., Boniforti L. et al. (1979) *J. Invest. Dermatol.* **73**, 126.
20. Jacobsen E., Billings J. K., Frantz R. A. et al. (1985) *J. Invest. Dermatol.* **85**, 483.
21. Harper W. F. and McNicol E. M. (1977) *Br. J. Dermatol.* **96**, 249.
22. Braverman I. M. Sibley J. and Keh-Yen A. (1986) *J. Invest. Dermatol.* **86**, 57.
23. Hull M. T. and Warfel K. A. (1983) *J. Invest. Dermatol.* **81**, 378.
24. Thuringer J. M. and Katzberg A. A. (1959) *J. Invest. Dermatol.* **33**, 35.
25. Baker H. and Blair C. P. (1968) *Br. J. Dermatol.* **80**, 367.
26. Epstein W. L. and Maibach H. I. (1965) *Arch. Dermatol.* **92**, 462.
27. Robbins J. H. and Moshell A. N. (1979) *J. Invest. Dermatol.* **73**, 102.
28. Liu S. C., Parsons S. and Hanawalt P. C. (1982) *J. Invest. Dermatol.* **79**, 330.
29. Gilchrest B. A. (1979) *J. Invest. Dermatol.* **72**, 219.
30. Gilchrest B. A., Szabo G., Flynn E. et al. (1983) *J. Invest. Dermatol.* **80**, 081S.
31. Marks R. (1981) *Br. J. Dermatol.* **104**, 627.
32. Plewig G. (1970) *J. Invest. Dermatol.* **54**, 19.
33. Potts R. O., Buras E. M. and Chrisman D. A. (1984) *J. Invest. Dermatol.* **82**, 97.
34. Daly C. H. and Odland G. F. (1979) *J. Invest. Dermatol.* **73**, 84.
35. Cronin E. (1980) *Contact Dermatitis.* Edinburgh, Churchill Livingstone, p. 21.
36. Coenraads P. J., Bleumink E. and Nater J. P. (1975) *Contact Dermatitis* **1**, 377.
37. Grove G. L., Lanker R. M., Hoelzle E. et al. (1982) *J. Soc. Cosmetic Chem.* **32**, 15.
38. Model D. (1985) *Br. Med. J.* **291**, 1755.
39. Grove G. L., Duncan S. and Kligman A. M. (1982) *Br. J. Dermatol.* **107**, 393.
40. Orentreich N., Markofsky J. and Vogelman J. H. (1979) *J. Invest. Dermatol.* **73**, 126.

7. CUTANEOUS INFECTIONS

N. H. Cox and D. T. Roberts

The types of cutaneous infection seen in elderly patients differ from those in younger patients for a variety of reasons. The most important of these is that diseases such as malignancy, diabetes, renal failure and poor nutrition are common in old age and predispose to infection. However, alterations in systemic immunity, and age-related changes in the skin and its bacterial flora are also of importance. Aspects of cutaneous ageing that may be of relevance to infection are discussed briefly, and cutaneous infections that are of particular importance in elderly patients are described.

AGE-RELATED CHANGES IN THE SKIN AND ITS BACTERIAL FLORA

Physiological changes in the skin secondary to ageing[1-3] include decreased activity of sebaceous and eccrine glands, the apocrine glands being largely unchanged. The antibacterial effect of substances such as free fatty acids in surface lipid may therefore be reduced. Both systemic and local cutaneous immune responsiveness decrease with increasing age.[1] Although the skin of elderly patients is often xerotic (partly due, in hospitals, to excessive washing), the intertriginous areas generally remain moist and harbour large numbers of aerobic organisms. Certain micro-organisms are more frequently isolated from the skin of the elderly than from other age-groups,[4] including streptococci (especially from the axillae) and *Candida albicans*. Enteric organisms are found in the toewebs of about one-fifth of elderly patients,[4] a fact that should be remembered when assessing the clinical importance of isolation of these organisms from leg ulcers.

BACTERIAL INFECTIONS

Furuncles and Carbuncles

Furuncles and carbuncles are deep infections of, respectively, a single hair follicle or contiguous group of follicles,[5,6] the causative organism being *Staphylococcus aureus*. Furuncles are most common in early adult life but carbuncles usually occur in middle-aged or elderly men.[5] Both are characterized by acute tenderness, erythema and swelling, with subsequent central necrosis. Symptoms due to carbuncles are more severe than those of furuncles, and fever and malaise are frequent. Carbuncles in particular are more frequent in patients with diabetes, malnutrition or poor general health, and in patients receiving long-term systemic steroid therapy. Treatment of furuncles depends on severity, but patients with a carbuncle require an appropriate systemic antibiotic (usually flucloxacillin, erythromycin or fusidic acid) after appropriate swabs have been obtained for bacterial culture. The advent of these drugs has led to established carbuncles becoming much less common than was previously the case. Patients who have recurrent lesions, in the absence of an underlying systemic disease, should be treated by eradication of staphylococci from carriage sites such as the anterior nares, umbilicus and flexures, plus regular washing with antiseptic soaps and the addition of antiseptics to the bath.

Erysipelas

Erysipelas is a superficial infection that may be severe and even fatal in elderly patients.[5] It is usually due to beta-haemolytic streptococci of Lancefield group A, and predisposing factors include diabetes, poor nutrition, alcoholism, haematological disorders and local oedema, especially of lymphatic or renal origin. It most commonly occurs on the face or feet, often with no obvious portal of entry (tinea pedis should be specifically excluded if recurrent episodes affect the feet). The face is becoming a less frequently affected site than the lower limbs and although there may be an increasing number of young patients affected, there remains a high prevalence among elderly diabetic patients. Erysipelas is characterized by rapid development of a well-demarcated, erythematous, infiltrated, tender plaque, sometimes with peripheral blistering. Occasionally, especially in the elderly, erysipelas may be haemorrhagic. Fever and systemic malaise are expected and may be severe. The diagnosis of erysipelas is made on the clinical features, as cultures are usually sterile and the ASO titre rises several days after the onset of symptoms. Prompt treatment with penicillin is required.

An important differential diagnosis in the elderly is an erysipelas-like erythema that can occur in elderly patients with diabetes.[7] In this disorder, well-demarcated areas of erythema develop on the lower leg similar in appearance to erysipelas but without pyrexia, leucocytosis or elevated ESR. The condition is precipitated by cardiac decompensation or unilateral venous thrombosis, and is accompanied by bony destruction in almost 40 per cent of patients.[8]

Cellulitis

Cellulitis is essentially the same process as erysipelas but occurring in the deeper connective tissues. It is usually due to streptococci, and there is commonly a portal of entry such as a wound or leg ulcer. The degree of erythema, swelling and tenderness is variable, and severe cases may be associated with constitutional symptoms, local bullae and regional lymphangitis and lymphadenopathy. In the elderly, decubitus and leg ulcers are a particularly important factor in the aetiology of cellulitis, which is suggested by a spreading rim of erythema around the ulcer. In such cases, it is important to identify the likely pathogen by bacterial cultures.

Bacterial Gangrene

Necrotizing fasciitis[9] (haemolytic streptococcal gangrene) and *progressive bacterial gangrene*[10] (Meleney's synergistic gangrene) are rare causes of cutaneous gangrene due to infection. The organisms implicated include haemolytic streptococci (probably the most important, especially in rapidly progressive gangrene), non-haemolytic microaerophilic streptococci, haemolytic staphylococci, diphtheroids, coliforms and *Pseudomonas*. Skin injury, either surgical or due to minor trauma, is an important part of the aetiology of these conditions, and both are most common in patients who are elderly, debilitated, diabetic, in cardiac failure, or who have peripheral vascular disease. Necrotizing fasciitis primarily affects the fascial layers superficial to muscle, skin necrosis being secondary to local vascular thrombosis, and is characterized by rapidly progressive cellulitis with dusky areas of necrosis, in patients who develop severe systemic toxicity. Progressive bacterial gangrene is less rapidly progressive, with less toxicity, but intermediate forms are frequent. There is a high mortality and prompt treatment is required. This includes surgical excision of affected tissue, antibiotics (a combination of benzyl penicillin, metronidazole and an aminoglycoside), nutritional support and correction of underlying diseases and the effects of systemic toxicity.

Leg Ulcers and Pressure Sores

Although primarily infective causes of leg ulceration are rare in elderly patients in the UK, secondary infection of gravitational and decubitus ulcers is a considerable problem. Bacterial colonization of such ulcers is universal, and the role of these bacteria in the progression of ulceration is a subject of debate. It is usual for ulcers below the waist to have a mixed flora, often including coliforms, *Pseudomonas* spp., staphylococci and streptococci. Coliforms are ubiquitous in the perineum and found in the toewebs of 20 per cent of elderly patients as a commensal, while *Pseudomonas* spp. are common in a hospital environment[11] and particularly inlongstanding ulcers because of their relative resistance to antiseptic agents. The clinical features are rarely helpful in identification of bacterial pathogens, but streptococcal infection may cause rapidly spreading cellulitis, *Pseudomonas* spp. are associated with bluish-green pus, *Pseudomonas putrefaciens* produces large amounts of hydrogen sulphide, and anaerobic organisms have a characteristic smell.

Even in the absence of overt cellulitis around an ulcer, a high bacterial load may be detrimental to healing. Ulcers with a bacterial count of over $10^5/cm^2$ did not heal in one study[12] but other authors did not demonstrate any correlation between bacterial colonization and healing of leg ulcers.[13] In spite of this disagreement, it seems prudent to use topical antiseptic agents as part of the management of decubitus and gravitational ulcers. Useful preparations with an antibacterial action include Eusol, Milton, benzoyl peroxide, hydrogen peroxide, silver nitrate, potassium permanganate and povidone-iodine. Topical antibiotics can be valuable in the treatment of leg ulcers, but their use should in general be short term because of the risk of local sensitization leading to development of allergic contact dermatitis with prolonged use. This is a particular problem with penicillins (not available for topical use), neomycin and framycetin. Silver sulphadiazine (Flamazine) is contra-indicated in patients allergic to sulphonamides but rarely causes local reactions. Chlortetracycline hydrochloride (Aureomycin) and mupirocin (Bactroban) are also unlikely to cause local hypersensitivity. Topical gentamicin is useful for ulcers infected with Gram-negative organisms, especially *Pseudomonas* spp., but widespread or long-term use of this agent may lead to development of resistant organisms and hence reduce the value of gentamicin for serious systemic infections. This argument also applies to the use of fusidic acid (Fucidin) for staphylococcal infections.

Bacterial counts from normal skin are greatly increased by occlusion with non-permeable dressings, but there are conflicting reports regarding the effect of modern biosynthetic dressings for treatment of ulcers on the bacterial flora. Some authors feel that these produce an environment conducive to the growth of bacteria,[14] while other studies have reported that the exudate under such dressings inhibits bacteria because it is acidic and contains viable neutrophil leucocytes.[15]

Malignant External Otitis

Malignant external otitis is due to infection of the external auditory canal by *Pseudomonas*.[16,17,18,19] It is a disease of elderly diabetic patients, and is infrequent in patients less than 55 years of age (9 per cent in a study of 34 cases).[18] It may be more frequent in patients who wear a hearing aid.[18] The clinical features, initially unilateral pain and purulent discharge, are due to cellulitis, osteitis, cranial nerve involvement (facial nerve in one-half of patients, cranial nerves VIII–XII in one-quarter) and meningitis (about 10 per cent). Aural polyps are found in most cases. Mortality is high and prompt treatment is required, consisting of surgical excision of affected tissue and systemic antibiotics.

Erythrasma

Erythrasma is a superfical skin infection due to *Corynebacterium minutissimum*. Infection of the toewebs is common and the organism may be part of the normal flora at this site. Clinical infection[5,6] usually involves the flexures, especially the genitocrural region, and is most common in a warm humid climate. Diabetes has been reported to be a risk factor.[20] Lesions are reddish-brown in colour, with dry skin and fine scaling, and are asymptomatic or only mildly pruritic. A simple test to confirm the diagnosis is to demonstrate the typical coral-red fluorescence of lesions when viewed with Wood's light, but skin scrapings should be taken for Gram staining (the preparations show Gram-positive rods, filaments and cocci) and to exclude dermatophyte infection. Treatment is with topical imidazole antifungals, Whitfield's ointment, or fusidic acid (Fucidin); alternatively, a 5-day course of oral erythromycin can be used.

Lupus Vulgaris

Lupus vulgaris (*Fig*. 7.1) is a form of cutaneous tuberculosis occurring as a post-primary infection in patients with a moderate or high degree of immunity.[21] It is rare, but still seen occasionally in elderly patients who may give a history of an enlarging cutaneous lesion of many years' duration. Lupus vulgaris is most commonly seen on the head and neck and is typically a reddish-brown, slowly enlarging, infiltrated plaque with some scaling and central scarring. The edge of the lesion consists of soft nodules with an 'apple-jelly' colour. Cartilage may be involved but bony destruction is rare. The diagnosis is made on the clinical and histopathological features, as the organism is rarely demonstrated in tissue sections or by culture methods. In this country, sarcoidosis, chronic discoid lupus erythematosus, syphilis and Bowen's disease are the most important differential diagnoses. Squamous cell carcinoma may develop in longstanding lesions of lupus vulgaris, and may present as an area of crusting or ulceration within an existing lesion of lupus vulgaris—such areas should therefore be biopsied to exclude malignant change. Treatment of lupus vulgaris is with a standard antituberculous drug regimen.

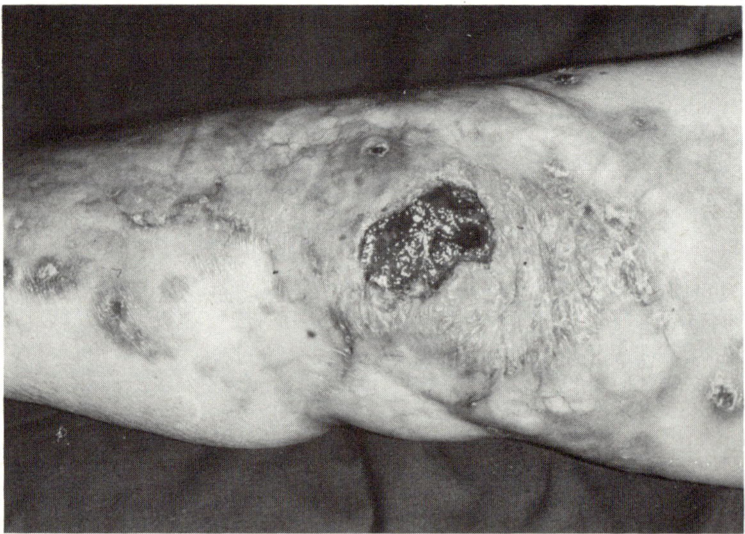

Fig. 7.1. Lupus vulgaris affecting the arm. The limbs are less frequently affected than the face. (Patient of Dr W. N. Morley.)

Tertiary Syphilis

Tertiary syphilis is rare now but cutaneous lesions are occasionally seen in elderly patients. The classical lesion is the gumma, which is a painless necrotic mass of syphilitic granulation tissue and usually presents as a punched-out ulcer or retracted scar. The scalp, central face, sternoclavicular region and tongue are the most commonly affected sites. Standard serological tests may be negative.

VIRAL INFECTIONS

Primary viral infections are rare in elderly patients. Warts are occasionally seen but are very uncommon and a solitary warty lesion is more likely to be a seborrhoeic wart (basal cell papilloma), actinic keratosis or squamous cell carcinoma. Herpes simplex in the elderly is usually due to reactivation of a 'cold sore' and the features are the same as in earlier adult life. Herpes zoster is discussed in detail as it is a cause of considerable morbidity in the elderly.

Herpes Zoster

Herpes zoster (shingles) affects 20 per cent of adults and is due to reactivation of the *Herpes varicella-zoster* virus, which remains latent in dorsal root ganglia after the primary infection (chickenpox). It is most common in the elderly and immunosuppressed,[22,23,24] with an incidence in the eighth decade 15 times that in the first decade of life. This is probably due to decreased immunological surveillance in the elderly.[25] The incidence of both ophthalmic involvement and post-herpetic neuralgia increases with increasing age, and local tissue damage is generally more severe in the elderly and immunosuppressed.

The typical clinical features are well knowm. Attacks may be triggered by surgery, trauma, irradiation, immunosuppression, malignancies, and infections such as tuberculosis, syphilis and malaria. Although the nerve most commonly affected is the trigeminal, the trunk is the most common site (about 50 per cent of cases involve dermatomes T3–L3) and a single dermatome is usually affected unilaterally. The names for the condition—*herpes* (Greek 'to creep'), *zoster* (Greek 'belt') and *shingles* (Latin *cingulus*, French *chingle*, both meaning 'belt' or 'girdle')—reflect the typical clinical pattern. The initial prodromal illness includes malaise, headache, fever, nausea and sometimes meningism. This is followed by burning and paraesthesiae in a dermatomal pattern with subsequent hyperaesthesia and local oedema and erythema. Vesicles develop that are initially clear, becoming yellow after about 3 days, crusted after 10 days and resolving in about 3–4 weeks. Pain may be severe in the elderly and patients with zoster affecting the sacral nerves may develop urinary retention (*Fig*. 7.2).

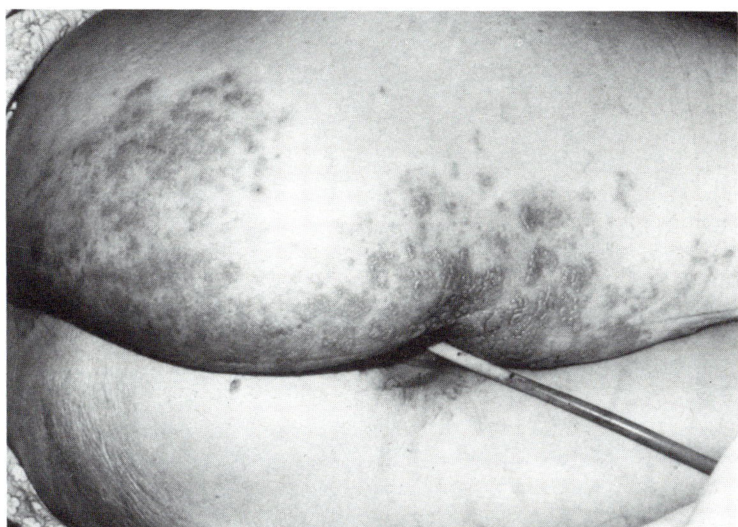

Fig. 7.2. Herpes zoster affecting the sacral nerves may cause severe pain and urinary retention. The rash is unilateral, with erythema and vesicles.

Extensive cutaneous necrosis may occur in elderly or immunosuppressed patients, but some patients in whom there is a brisk amnestic response may develop neuralgia without subsequent vesiculation (zoster *sine herpete*).[26] Although a few vesicles outside the affected dermatome are commonly found due to haematogenous spread, more than 10 aberrant vesicles suggests true disseminated disease that may be both cutaneous (varicella-like) and visceral. This occurs in 2–10 per cent of patients, especially those who are elderly, immunosupressed or who have ocular involvement.

Herpes zoster opthhalmicus warrants special mention as it is a particular problem of the elderly.[27] Involvement of the nasociliary nerve, which causes vesicles on the tip of the nose (Hutchinson's sign), occurs in one-third of patients with herpes zoster ophthalmicus and is a predictor of ophthalmic involvement. Some form of ocular involvement may occur in over two-thirds of patients with herpes zoster ophthalmicus,[28] including lid ulceration and scarring, proptosis, ptosis and ocular palsies, conjunctivitis, uveitis, corneal abnormalities (oedema, keratitis, vesiculation, ulceration, lipid deposition, vascularization, anaesthesia and abrasion), and occasionally acute retinal necrosis. Post-herpetic neuralgia is common in elderly patients with ophthalmic nerve involvement, affecting 50 per cent of patients aged over 60 years.

Herpes zoster affecting the maxillary division of the trigeminal nerve causes vesicles on the uvula and tonsillar region, and vesicles occur on the tongue, floor of the mouth and buccal mucosa when the mandibular division of the trigeminal nerve is involved. In the Ramsay Hunt syndrome, severe pain in the ear is followed by facial paralysis and development of vesicles in the external auditory canal, on the pinna and over the mastoid process—this may be accompanied by facial or palatal sensory loss due to involvement of the Vth and IXth cranial nerves respectively.

The diagnosis is often clear clinically, but the virus may be demonstrated by electron microscopy or immunofluorescent staining of vesicle fluid, scrapings or Tzank smears from the base of vesicles, or biopsy specimens. A rise in antibody titre on serology will retrospectively confirm the diagnosis.

Antiviral agents should be used to treat herpes zoster in the first week but are of no value after this time. Acyclovir is indicated for treatment of herpes zoster in immunosuppressed patients and for patients with recurrent or disseminated zoster. It will decrease acute pain but does not appear to reduce the incidence of post-herpetic neuralgia[29]—the oral preparation does not reliably exceed the LD_{50} for the varicella-zoster virus and the drug should therefore be administered intravenously. For topical application, idoxuridine 5 per cent or 40 per cent in dimethylsulphoxide (DMSO) should be applied every

4–6 hours. Although some authors argue that systemic or topical steroids may increase dissemination of the virus, there is evidence that they can decrease pain[29,30] and ocular complications,[30] and that high-dose systemic steroids may reduce the incidence of post-herpetic neuralgia.[29]

FUNGAL INFECTIONS

Candida Infections

Candida infections of the skin are usually due to *Candida albicans*, which is a normal commensal of the gastrointestinal tract and some skin sites. Although the incidence of candidosis is high in old age, some authorities feel that this is due to the diseases and treatments associated with old age, rather than with increasing age *per se*.[31] Factors predisposing to clinical infection include antibiotic therapy, systemic steroid therapy, immunosuppression, debilitating disease, and local cutaneous factors such as maceration, moisture and trauma. The prevalence of oral yeasts rises in old age[32] but that of vaginal yeasts falls after the menopause.

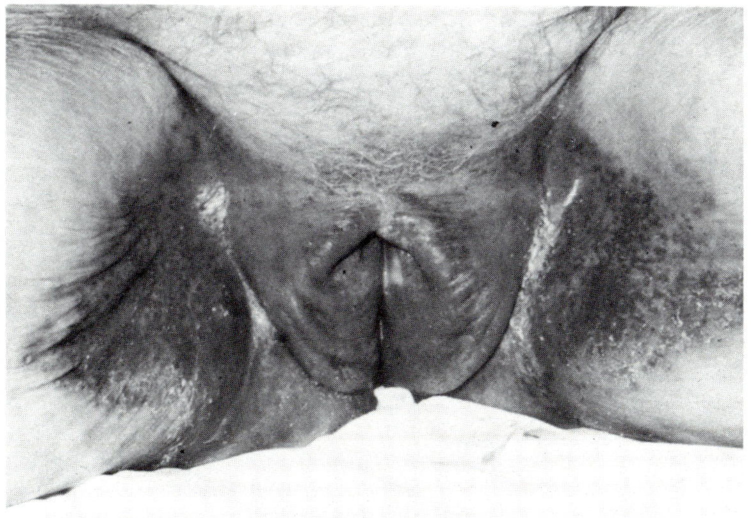

Fig. 7.3. Candidal intertrigo. Moist macerated skin is commonly affected.

Cutaneous candidosis[31,33] typically involves the axillae, groins and inframammary regions, especially in obese patients and if the skin is moist and macerated (*Fig.* 7.3). It is a common problem in elderly patients in hospital. Affected areas are a beefy red colour with satellite lesions outside the border of the main lesion. The satellite lesions consist of papules, pustules (often follicular) and erosions, and these are also seen at the edge of the main lesion. Between the toes, and in the fingerwebs (erosio interdigitalis blastomycetica), the skin becomes thickened, white and fissured, without satellite lesions. Treatment is with astringent soaks to dry the affected area, and nystatin- or imidazole-containing antifungal creams (often combined with 1 per cent hydrocortisone to reduce inflammation, e.g. Daktacort). Subsequent prophylactic measures include weight reduction, thorough local washing and drying daily, and regular use of talc dusting powders. Underlying systemic disease predisposing to candidosis should also be treated.

Angular cheilitis in the elderly is often due to candida infection, although other infections can cause the same appearance, and iron deficiency may be a cause. Angular cheilitis due to *Candida albicans* infection (perlèche) usually occurs in association with either denture stomatitis or oral thrush[31] and is common in the elderly because loss of facial height associated with edentia or with the wearing of worn dentures causes deep folds to develop at the angles of the mouth.[34] Treatment is with topical nystatin, amphotericin B or an imidazole, with concurrent treatment of the mouth using nystatin suspension or amphotericin B lozenges. Dentures should be thoroughly cleaned, removed each night (and soaked in a cleansing agent such as Milton), and nystatin or amphotericin B cream should be applied to the fitting surface before use.

Oral candidosis may present as several different clinical entities.[31,33,35] These are oral rather than cutaneous infections but are listed because of the association with angular cheilitis. Denture stomatitis (denture sore mouth) is the commonest and is seen in 60 per cent of denture wearers over the age of 65 years.[36] Other conditions include acute pseudomembranous candidosis (thrush), acute atrophic candidosis (including 'antibiotic sore tongue'), candida leukoplakia and central papillary atrophy of the tongue (median rhomboid glossitis).

Dermatophyte Infections (Ringworm)

Dermatophyte infections (ringworm) are comparatively unusual in elderly patients. Ringworm of the scalp is seen in children, and ringworm of the feet or groin in young adults. Ringworm of the body (tinea corporis) can affect any age, but extensive infections are more frequent in patients who are debilitated or immunosuppressed. Dermatophyte infection of the palms and of the nails warrants further discussion as this may be a chronic problem.

Dermatophyte infection of the palms is usually due to *Trichophyton rubrum* and is often a longstanding problem.[37] It is usually unilateral, in contrast to hand dermatitis, and causes few symptoms. The palm appears erythematous with fine white scaling in the palmar creases. Skin scrapings should always be taken to confirm the diagnosis as topical treatment is unlikely to be effective, the majority of patients requiring at least 6 weeks of oral griseofulvin (1 g daily with a meal).

Tinea unguium, dermatophyte infection of the nails, is often suspected in elderly patients although only about 15 per cent of nail dystrophies are due to fungal infection.[38] Thickening of the hallux nails is extremely common in elderly patients but may have other causes such as peripheral vascular disease. The commonest type of tinea unguium causes distal thickening and discoloration (usually yellowish-brown) of affected nails, other nails appearing normal. As treatment involves 12–18 months of oral griseofulvin, with a less than 50 per cent success rate, it is essential that the diagnosis is confirmed by mycological examination of nail clippings before starting therapy. The decision to commence therapy should be taken with the poor success rate in mind. Although treatment is usually recommended in some patients (for example, diabetics), many asymptomatic patients may elect not to have treatment. Topical therapy alone will not effect a cure, but it may be a useful adjunct to chemical removal of the nail using urea ointment.

INFESTATIONS

Scabies

Scabies is not common over the age of 50 years but can occur in outbreaks in nursing homes and geriatric medicine departments,[39,40] and is often misdiagnosed because the clinical picture is dominated by non-specific excoriations and secondary infection. The cardinal symptom is itch, usually worse at night, and usually severe. Burrows containing the scabies mite and eggs are most commonly found in the fingerwebs, on the volar wrists and ulnar border of the hands, on the extensor aspect of the elbows, around the nipples, in the natal cleft and umbilicus, and on the penis. Vesicles may be found at some of these sites. Small erythematous papular 'secondary lesions', probably due to allergic sensitization, occur at other sites such as the trunk and buttocks, and are also extremely itchy. Norwegian scabies is a highly contagious form of scabies in which an impaired host response allows heavy infestation with mites. Patients are usually mentally deficient, elderly and debilitated, or immunosuppressed. Itch may be severe, and the clinical findings are gross hyperkeratosis of hands and feet, thickened nails, and extensive areas of scaling erythema of the head, neck and trunk. The diagnosis may first be suspected when other patients or staff develop more typical 'ordinary' scabies. The crusted lesions of patients with Norwegian scabies contain huge numbers of mites, and attendant medical and nursing staff may easily develop infestation.

Several preparations are available for treatment, such as gamma benzene hexachloride 0·1 per cent, and monosulfiram. Benzyl benzoate can also be used but is irritant. It is important to treat contacts at the same time, including medical and nursing staff, in order to prevent reinfection. It should also be realized that itch and inflammatory nodules may persist for several weeks after perfectly adequate treatment, and can be treated with a topical steroid. Persistent itch is not an indication for retreatment, unless mites can still be demonstrated, as this may lead to irritant contact dermatitis and therefore perpetuate itch and dermatitic rash.

Lice

Lice are most common in vagrants, and infrequent changing of clothes, low intellect, poor health and malnutrition are all predisposing factors.[41] Treatment should include thorough disinfestation of clothing as lice and eggs are likely to be most numerous in the seams of clothing adjacent to the skin.

REFERENCES

1. Gilchrest B. A. (1984) *Skin and Aging Processes.* Boca Raton, Florida, CRC Press, p. 26.
2. Silver A., Montagna W. and Karacon I. (1964) *J. Invest. Dermatol.* **43**, 255.
3. Montagna W. (1959) *J. Invest. Dermatol.* **33**, 151.
4. Somerville D. A. (1969) *Br. J. Dermatol.* **81** (Suppl. 1), 14.
5. Roberts S. O. B. and Rook A. (1979) In: Rook A., Wilkinson D. S. and Ebling F. J. G. (eds) *Textbook of Dermatology*, 3rd ed. Oxford, Blackwell Scientific, p. 541.
6. Maibach H. I. and Hacker P. (1975) In: Moschella S. L., Pillsbury D. M. and Hurley H. H. (eds) *Dermatology*. Philadelphia, W. B. Saunders Company, p. 491.
7. Lithner F. (1974) *Acta Med. Scand.* **196**, 333.
8. Lithner F. and Hietala S.-O. (1976) *Acta Med. Scand.* **200**, 155.
9. Rea W. J. and Wyrick W. J. (1970) *Ann. Surg.* **172**, 957.
10. Ledingham I. and Tehrani M. A. (1975) *Br. J. Surg.* **62**, 364.
11. Noble W. C. and White P. M. (1969) *Trans. St Johns Hosp. Dermatol. Soc.* **55**, 202.
12. Lookingbill D. P., Miller S. H. and Knowles R. C. (1978) *Arch. Dermatol.* **114**, 1765.
13. Eriksson G. (1985) In: Ryan T. J. (ed.) *An Environment for Healing: The Role of Occlusion. R. Soc. Med. Int. Congr. Symp. Ser.* No. 88. London, Royal Society of Medicine, p. 45.
14. Katz S., McGinley K. and Leyden J. L. (1986) *Arch. Dermatol.* **122**, 58.
15. Varghese M. C., Balin A. K., Carter D. M. et al. (1986) *Arch. Dermatol.* **122**, 52.
16. Wilson D. F., Pulec J. L. and Linthicum F. H. (1971) *Arch. Otolaryngol.* **93**, 419.
17. Petrozzi J. W. and Warthan T. L. (1974) *Arch. Dermatol.* **110**, 258.

18. Zaky D. A., Bentley D. W., Lowy K. et al. (1976) *Am. J. Med.* **61**, 298.
19. Salit I. E., McNeely D. J. and Chait G. (1985) *Can. Med. Assoc. J.* **132**, 381.
20. Montes L. F., Dobson H., Dodge B. G. et al. (1969) *Arch. Dermatol.* **99**, 674.
21. Wilkinson D. S. (1979) In: Rook A., Wilkinson D. S. and Ebling F. J. G. (eds) *Textbook of Dermatology*, 3rd ed. Oxford, Blackwell Scientific, p. 677.
22. Editorial. (1979) *Br. Med. J.* **i**, 5.
23. Weller T. (1983) *N. Engl. J. Med.* **309**, 1362, 1434.
24. Liesegang T. J. (1984) *J. Am. Acad. Dermatol.* **11**, 165.
25. Berger R., Florent G. and Just M. (1981) *Infect. Immunol.* **32**, 24.
26. Easton H. G. (1970) *Lancet* **ii**, 1065.
27. Rogers R. S. and Tindall J. P. (1971) *J. Am. Geriatr. Soc.* **19**, 495.
28. Womack L. W. and Liesegang T. J. (1983) *Arch. Ophthalmol.* **101**, 42.
29. Stewart J. C. M., Ferguson J. and Davey P. (1983) *Br. Med. J.* **286**, 1802.
30. Scheie H. G. (1970) *Trans. Ophthalmol. Soc. UK* **90**, 899.
31. Odds F. C. (1979) *Candida and Candidosis*. Leicester, Leicester University Press, pp. 78, 96, 113.
32. Smits B. J., Prior A. P. and Arblaster P. G. (1966) *Br. Med. J.* **i**, 208.
33. DeCastro P. and Jorizzo J. L. (1985) *Semin. Dermatol.* **4**, 165.
34. Chernosky M. E. (1966) *Arch. Dermatol.* **93**, 332.
35. Tyldesley W. R. (1981) *Oral Medicine*. Oxford, Oxford University Press, p. 32.
36. Budtz-Jorgensen E., Stenderup A. and Grabowski M. (1975) *Community Dent. Oral Epidemiol.* **3**, 115.
37. Roberts S. O. B. and MacKenzie D. W. R. (1979) In: Rook A., Wilkinson D. S. and Ebling F. J. G. (eds) *Textbook of Dermatology*, 3rd ed. Oxford, Blackwell Scientific, p. 767.
38. Roberts D. T. and Tuyp E. (1985) *Semin. Dermatol.* **4**, 222.
39. Herridge C. F. (1963) *Br. Med. J.* **i**, 239.
40. Moberg S. A. W., Löwhagen G. E. and Hersle K. S. (1984) *J. Am. Acad. Dermatol.* **11**, 242.
41. Alexander J. O'D. *Arthropods and Human Skin*. Berlin, Springer-Verlag, pp. 45–46.

8. BLISTERING DISEASES IN OLD AGE

Anne P. Harrison and N. B. Simpson

Blisters occur in many skin diseases and at all ages. Often there are known causes such as allergic contact sensitization, exposure to chemical irritants, infection (bacterial, fungal, viral, parasitic), vascular occlusion or physical injury (heat, cold, ionizing radiation, ultraviolet light, mechanical trauma). This chapter concentrates on those diseases of the elderly that are primarily bullous in nature.

The clinical features are determined by the site of the lesion within the skin. Therefore, before further discussion of these conditions it may be helpful to recall the structure of the epidermis and some aspects of dermo-epidermal interaction. Light microscopy delineates four layers: (1) the basal layer resting on the basal lamina, which is in contact with the dermis; (2) the spinous cell layer; (3) the granular layer; (4) the horny layer. Electron microscopy shows that the basal lamina is separated from the membrane of the basal cell by a less dense zone—the lamina lucida. Short striated anchoring fibrils bind the lamina lucida to the dermis. The epidermis is composed of keratinocytes and the cohesive strength of the normal epidermis depends on the integrity of desmosomes between these cells. Following damage to this functional region there is loss of intercellular adhesion and the keratinocytes round off and separate. This is termed 'acantholysis'.[1]

The basic locations of blister formation are: (1) intra-epidermal—producing flaccid, easily ruptured blisters as in pemphigus, and (2) subepidermal—producing tense blisters as in pemphigoid, dermatitis herpetiformis, porphyria cutanea tarda and erythema multiforme. Histological distinctions can be deceptive as the basal layer of the epidermis and basement membrane may be re-established in as little as 24 hours in subepidermal bullae to give the erroneous appearance of an intra-epidermal split. Therefore, biopsy should only be performed on fresh blisters (less than 24 hours old). In addition to histological assessment it is important to consider the clinical appearance and history, the immunological findings and response to treatment when forming a diagnosis. The rest of this chapter consists of a discussion of the more common blistering diseases encountered in the practice of medicine in the elderly.

PEMPHIGUS

Pemphigus vulgaris is the commonest and most serious type of pemphigus. It occurs predominantly in the middle-aged and elderly. In over 50 per cent of cases the disease begins with painful erosions in the mouth and may persist there for some months before skin involvement;[2] other mucous membranes may be similarly affected. Clinically, flaccid blisters or superficial erosions, which look like scalds, develop on the trunk and head.

Histologically, acantholysis is the hallmark of pemphigus.[3] Pemphigus IgG auto-antibodies bind to a surface antigen on squamous epithelial cells and induce cell-to-cell detachment and acantholysis.[4] Direct immunofluorescence demonstrates IgG antibody deposits in intercellular spaces in perilesional skin.[5] A circulating IgG antibody can be detected in the serum of 70–90 per cent of patients by indirect immunofluorescence.[6] Serum or IgG fractions from pemphigus patients can induce acantholysis in cultures of human skin explants.[4] A pemphigus-like disease has been induced in neonatal mice by IgG fractions.[7] The interaction of IgG auto-antibody with epidermal cell surface antigen causes synthesis or activation of a non-lysosomal proteolytic enzyme (pemphigus activation factor), which may be plasminogen activator,[8] and may lead to hydrolysis at the cell surface and loss of intercellular adhesion.[9] The role of complement remains obscure but recent work suggests that it may have a very important function in altering the integrity of the cell membrane in the presence of antibody.[10] There is a significant relationship between disease activity and serum antibody titre at presentation. However, serial titres are too inconsistent to be used as indicators of prognosis or efficacy of therapy.[11]

The other forms of pemphigus are rarely encountered. Pemphigus foliaceous is a less serious form of pemphigus in which lesions remain localized. Acantholysis occurs in the high intra-epidermal region. Pemphigus erythematosus shows some features of pemphigus foliaceous and some immunological features of lupus erythematosus. It is a localized disorder and can be managed by topical corticosteroid treatment alone. Pemphigus may be associated with other autoimmune disorders, thymoma and myasthenia gravis.[12] Penicillamine and captopril may induce pemphigus vulgaris or foliaceous, which may then progress to established disease on withdrawal of the drug.[9]

In the pre-steroid era, most patients with severe pemphigus died of their disease; today, high-dose corticosteroids and intensive nursing care have greatly improved the outlook for sufferers of this disease. Most drug regimens involve a daily starting dose of prednisolone of 100 mg or more with early introduction of either azathioprine or cyclophosphamide as 'steroid sparing agents'. Occasionally doses as high as 400 mg prednisolone/day are required to induce remission. Therapy may have to be continued for many years but eventually the disease 'burns out' in those patients who survive the effects of treatment.[13,14] Topical steroids and antistaphylococcal antibiotics are often useful adjuncts.[15]

BULLOUS PEMPHIGOID

Bullous pemphigoid is a disease of the elderly, 80 per cent of cases occurring in patients over the age of 60 years. In general it is less serious than pemphigus although if extensive it may be life threatening. Spontaneous resolution may occur after 5–6 years.[16] Onset may be sudden but some patients suffer from prolonged pruritus before the diagnosis is made.[17] Large, tense, often haemorrhagic blisters appear on normal skin and one-third of patients develop oral blisters.[16]

Histolologically, the bullae are subepidermal with an eosinophilic and neutrophilic infiltrate in the upper dermis. Typically deposits of IgG and C3 are found in the lamina lucida of perilesional skin although other immunoglobulins and complement may also be seen.[18] A circulating basement membrane zone antibody can be found in 50–70 per cent of patients, but while this can be a useful diagnostic test, it is a poor indicator of disease activity. Indeed, it has been difficult to demonstrate the pathogenic action of circulating bullous pemphigoid antibodies.[18] Subclassification of the auto-antibody shows an increase in IgG4 which, although non-complement fixing, is thought to have homocytotrophic properties for mast cells. It is possible that following antigen–antibody contact in the skin, mast cells are bound and provoked to degranulate, thus releasing chemotactic factors for eosinophils and neutrophils. Release of proteolytic enzymes may then result in cleavage of the dermo-epidermal junction.[19]

The often quoted association between bullous pemphigoid and malignancy remains controversial.[20] Overall there is no statistically significant association, the common factor being increased age, and the association is one of coincidence.[12] Some studies suggest that concurrent malignancy is more common in those patients who fail to demonstrate indirect immunofluorescence of perilesional skin. Mucosal involvement is more common in the seronegative group.[20]

The disease is usually brought under control with moderately high doses of corticosteroids (prednisolone 80–100 mg/day). In general the older the patient the better the response to treatment. There are potential dangers in the use of such high steroid doses; congestive cardiac failure, diabetes mellitus or steroid psychoses may be precipitated in the elderly patient. These effects may be minimized by starting therapy with azathioprine to reduce the requirement for steroids.

However, immunosuppressants should be used with caution in this age-group because of the likelihood of occult malignancy. It is usually possible to reduce the steroid dose within a few weeks and maintain the patient on 10–15 mg prednisolone daily with further cautious reduction thereafter. Plasma exchange is an effective means of lowering steroid requirements, but despite disease control it has not found widespread acceptance because of cost, availability and the potential hazard of fluid overload in the elderly patient.[21]

CICATRICIAL PEMPHIGOID (BENIGN MUCOUS MEMBRANE PEMPHIGOID)

Cicatricial pemphigoid belies its alternative name because it is a most distressing disease of the elderly. The average age of onset is 50–65 years and it follows a chronic scarring course with a predilection for mucosal surfaces and little tendency to remission.[22] The most commonly involved sites, in order of frequency, are: oral mucosa, conjunctivae, larynx, genitalia and oesophagus. In one-third of cases there may be skin involvement consisting of short-lived, scattered, tense, non-scarring bullae in flexures or around the umbilicus, or alternatively one or more erythematous areas that blister recurrently and ultimately scar.[23] One form, known as the Brunsting Perry type, is manifest by recurrent blisters on the head and neck with sparing of the mucous membranes.[24] The subepidermal blisters are characteristic and deposits of IgA and C3 are found in the lamina lucida. Circulating antibodies to the basement membrane zone have been sought but found only infrequently.[25]

Stricture and scar formation resulting in near blindness or gradual oesophageal or laryngeal obstruction may occur. High-dose prednisolone is usually prescribed,[26] but is rarely helpful. Immunosuppressants, dapsone and cytotoxic drugs have had similarly disappointing results. Symptomatic relief with powerful topical steroids for the skin and the oral and pharyngeal mucous membranes is often the best that can be hoped for.

DERMATITIS HERPETIFORMIS

Dermatitis herpetiformis (DH) is a chronic, intensely itchy, bullous skin disease with a biphasic pattern of incidence, the first peak being in young adults and the second in the elderly. The cutaneous eruption has a characteristic distribution of small blisters affecting the extensor surfaces of limbs, buttocks, shoulders, axillary folds and scalp. Diagnosis can be confirmed by biopsy of an early lesion that shows, on light microscopy, collections of polymorphs at the tips of the dermal papillae.

Direct immunofluorescence of involved and non-involved skin shows the pathognomonic features of granular deposits of IgA and complement components C3 and C5 at the tips of the dermal papillae. Up to 15 per cent of patients may show a linear, band-like deposition of IgA at the dermo-epidermal junction.[27] This group is called 'linear IgA disease' (*see below*).

Dermatitis herpetiformis responds rapidly to dapsone in a dosage of 50–150 mg/day. The lowest dose possible should be used to avoid the complications of methaemoglobinaemia and haemolytic anaemia. Sulphapyridine is an alternative but less frequently used treatment. The rapid clinical response to dapsone may be useful in confirming the diagnosis. Eighty per cent of patients with DH have HLA-B8[28] and even more (80–100 per cent) have an associated gluten-sensitive enteropathy (GSE).[27,29,30] Clinical features of GSE may be absent but a gluten-free diet can be useful in control of the disease and can reduce the requirement for dapsone.[31] There have been multiple reports of lymphoma of the small intestine in DH patients with GSE and this should be considered in any patients who have unexplained abdominal symptoms.[12] Linear IgA disease can be separated from the granular IgA type of DH by the absence of associated GSE and HLA-B8.[27] However, the former responds poorly to dapsone but may be treated successfully with sulphapyridine.

PORPHYRIA CUTANEA TARDA

Porphyria cutanea tarda (PCT) is a metabolic disorder of haem biosynthesis that results in a distinctive pattern of excess porphyrin production and cutaneous manifestations. The disease was formerly thought to be acquired and related to alcoholic liver disease but a specific inheritable enzyme defect in the haem biosynthetic pathway has been indentified.[32,33] Deficiency in the activity of the enzyme uroporphyrinogen decarboxylase is the primary defect but interaction with external factors such as alcohol, oestrogens or iron overload is usually required for the full clinical expression of the disease. The enzyme deficiency results in the accumulation of 8- to 5-carboxylic porphyrinogens that are oxidized to form photoactive porphyrin byproducts.

The cutaneous manifestations are variable but usually include skin fragility, vesicles and blisters, hyperpigmentation, hypertrichosis, scarring alopecia, onycholysis and sclerodermoid skin change. Light-exposed areas of the face, dorsum of the hands and arms are predominantly affected. Histology of a vesicular lesion shows a subepidermal bulla. Clinical diagnosis is confirmed by finding a consistent porphyrin profile in blood, faeces and urine. In PCT the urinary uroporphyrin to coproporphyrin ratio is usually greater than 4 : 1. In all cases there is associated liver disease, which may be mild, but cirrhosis, hepatitis and hepatoma do occur. An association with lupus erythematosus has been noted and this is of importance in considering appropriate therapy for either condition.[12]

BULLOUS DRUG ERUPTIONS

The elderly patient is likely to take a large number of drugs capable of producing rashes and blisters but it is outside the scope of this chapter to discuss these in detail. Barbiturates, iodine, bromides and sulphonamides can cause blisters. Phenolphthalein may give rise to a fixed drug eruption and nalidixic acid a bullous photosensitization. This cause of blistering should be evident from the history.

BULLOUS ERYTHEMA MULTIFORME

This eruption is commonly associated with herpes simplex, mycoplasma infection and drug ingestion although other reported associations are legion. The typical appearance is of a 'target' lesion found on the hands, feet and extensor aspects of the limbs, but frank blistering may also occur in these sites or occasionally on mucous membranes. Severe skin and mucous membrane involvement with constitutional upset and a significant mortality is known as the Stevens–Johnson syndrome. Many textbooks recommend systemic steroids for severe erythema multiforme but in our experience symptomatic treatment with local antiseptics is usually all that is necessary. Recurrent erythema multiforme is a very troublesome condition and is often triggered by herpes simplex infection, in which case topical application of idoxuridine or acyclovir to the cold sore may prevent the development of erythema multiforme.

ADULT TOXIC EPIDERMAL NECROLYSIS

This is often of sudden onset with severe constitutional upset. Although considered to be a severe variety of erythema multiforme by some, this relationship remains controversial. There is a bullous phase of the condition followed by lysis of the superficial epidermis and extensive mucous membrane involvement. It has been associated with phenylbutazone, barbiturates, sulphonamides, phenolphthalein, hydantoin, post radiotherapy and in association with lymphomas. Mortality may be as high as 50 per cent and intensive supportive therapy as for a severe burn is necessary.

BULLOUS ERUPTION OF DIABETICS

This eruption occurs on the hands and feet of diabetics and may be related to disturbed carbohydrate metabolism, although failure to control the diabetes or the presence of peripheral neuropathy is not significantly associated. There is often an accompanying microvasculopathy. The blisters are subepidermal or intra-epidermal and direct immunofluorescence is generally negative.[31,34]

BULLAE COMPLICATING CEREBRAL DAMAGE

Bullae have been described following cerebrovascular catastrophe. Blisters are not necessarily on pressure areas but do occur on hemiplegic limbs and are indicative of a poor prognosis.[35]

BULLOUS DISEASE OF DIALYSIS

Acquired subepidermal blisters in association with haemodialysis for chronic renal failure usually occur on exposed skin. There is photosensitivity but the aetiology is obscure. Porphyrin metabolism is normal and there is no constant relationship with frusemide treatment. The condition is generally self-limiting but sun avoidance may be helpful.

EPIDERMOLYSIS BULLOSA ACQUISITA

This condition occurs in adult life and is really a dermolytic disease. There is clinical, histological and immunohistological overlap with bullous pemphigoid and cicatricial pemphigoid but there are specific differences. Clinically, bullae develop over the joints of the hands, feet, elbows and knees following minor trauma and result in atrophic scarring and milia.[36] However, some patients have little evidence of milia, scarring or traumatic lesions.[37]

Histologically the split occurs below the basal lamina and distinguishes epidermolysis bullosa acquisita from bullous pemphigoid or cicatricial pemphigoid. A dense granular material staining for IgG is found at the basement membrane zone.[38] There is a strong association with systemic diseases such as inflammatory bowel disease, lymphoma, myeloma, systemic lupus erythematosus, carcinoma of the bronchus or pulmonary fibrosis, and drugs such as frusemide, sulphonamides and penicillamine have also been implicated. It is suggested that these conditions or drugs result in the production of an antibody directed towards a specific basement membrane zone protein, which binds beneath the lamina lucida.[39] The condition is relatively resistant to steroid therapy and management is difficult.

SUMMARY

Bullous diseases are common. The clinical characteristics are misleading; a careful history may eliminate drug-related and metabolic causes. A full examination of the entire skin and mucous membranes is mandatory for all patients and skin biopsy with immunofluorescence is often necessary to establish the diagnosis.

REFERENCES

1. McKie R. M. (ed.) (1984) *Milne's Dermatopathology*, 2nd ed. London, Edward Arnold.
2. Bean S. F., Fritz K. A. and Jordan R. E. (1984) *J. Am. Acad. Dermatol.* **11**, 1151.
3. Civatte A. (1943) *Ann. Dermatol. Syphilol. (Paris)* **3**, 1.
4. Anhalt G. J., Patel H. and Diaz L. A. (1983) *Arch. Dermatol.* **119**, 711.
5. Beutner E. H. and Jordan R. E. (1964) *Proc. Soc. Exp. Biol. Med.* **117**, 505.
6. Beutner E. H., Lever W. F., Witebsky E. et al. (1965) *J. Am. Acad. Dermatol.* **192**, 682.
7. Peterson L. L. and Wuepper K. D. (1983) *Clin. Res.* **31**, 569A.
8. Skerrow C. J. (1985) *J. Dermatol.* **113**, 765.
9. Thiers B. H. (1981) *J. Am. Acad. Dermatol.* **4**, 603.
10. Kawana S., Geoghegan W. D. and Jordan R. E. (1986) *J. Invest. Dermatol.* **86**, 29.
11. Fitzpatrick R. E. and Newcomer V. D. (1980) *Arch. Dermatol.* **116**, 285.
12. Callen J. P. (1980) *J. Am. Acad. Dermatol.* **3**, 10.
13. Ryan J. G. (1971) *Arch. Dermatol.* **104**, 14.
14. Rosenberg F. R., Sanders S. and Nelson C. T. (1976) *Arch. Dermatol.* **112**, 962.
15. Levene G. M. (1982) *Clin. Exp. Dermatol.* **7**, 643.
16. Lever W. F. (1979) *J. Am. Acad. Dermatol.* **1**, 2.
17. Bingham E. A., Burrows D. and Sandford J. C. (1984) *Clin. Exp. Dermatol.* **9**, 564.
18. Thiers B. H. (1982) *J. Am. Acad. Dermatol.* **6**, 1103.
19. Bird P., Friedman P. S., Ling N. et al (1986) *J. Invest. Dermatol.* **86**, 21.
20. Hodge L., Marsden R. A., Black M. M. et al. (1981) *Br. J. Dermatol.* **105**, 65.
21. Roujeau J. C., Guillame J. C., Morel P. et al. (1984) *Lancet* **ii**, 486.
22. Person J. R. and Rogers R. S., 3rd (1977) *Mayo Clin. Proc.* **52**, 54.
23. Hardy K. M., Perry H. O., Pingree G. C. et al. (1971) *Arch. Dermatol.* **104**, 467.
24. Brunsting L. A. and Perry H. O. (1957) *Arch. Dermatol.* **75**, 489.
25. Fine J.-D., Neises G. R. and Katz S. I. (1984) *J. Invest. Dermatol.* **82**, 39.
26. Schmitz R. and Hautkr Z. (1958) *Z. Haut. Geschlechtskr.* **28**, 36.
27. Fry L. and Seah P. P. (1974) *Br. J. Dermatol.* **90**, 137.
28. Lawley T. J., Strober W., Yaoita M. D. et al. (1980) *J. Invest. Dermatol.* **74**, 9.
29. Buckley D. B., English J., Molloy W. et al. (1983) *Clin. Exp. Dermatol.* **8**, 477.
30. Fry L., Seah P. P., McMinn R. M. H. et al. (1972) *Br. Med. J.* **3**, 371.
31. Epstein W. L., Katz S. I., Sams W. M. et al. (1984) *J. Am. Acad. Dermatol.* **11**, 1151.
32. Kushner J. P. and Barbato A. J. (1975) *Clin. Res.* **23**, 403A.
33. Kushner J. P., Barbato A. J. and Lee G. R. (1976) *J. Clin. Invest.* **58**, 1089.
34. Allen G. E. and Hadden D. R. (1970) *Br. J. Dermatol.* **82**, 216.
35. Paltzik R. L. (1980) *Arch. Dermatol.* **116**, 475.
36. Roenick H. H., Ryan J. G. and Bergfield W. F. (1971) *Arch. Dermatol.* **103**, 1.
37. Gammon W. R., Briggaman R. A., Woodley D. T. et al. (1984) *J. Am. Acad. Dermatol.* **11**, 820.
38. Palestine R. F., Kossard S. and Dicken C. H. (1981) *J. Am. Acad. Dermatol.* **5**, 43.
39. Yaoita H., Briggaman R. A., Lawley T. J. et al. (1981) *J. Invest. Dermatol.* **76**, 288.

9. CUTANEOUS MALIGNANCY IN OLD AGE

Rona M. MacKie

A large number of benign, pre-malignant and malignant tumours arise from both the epidermis and the dermis. This of course reflects the wide range of cells that are found within the skin. With very few exceptions, benign, pre-malignant and malignant cutaneous tumours are found more frequently in those over the age of 60 than in those under the age of 30. Interesting exceptions to this include the benign viral wart, the benign melanocytic naevus and the basal cell carcinoma arising on the basis of an organoid or sebaceous naevus.

It would appear from the first of these three observations that the skin of the elderly is less susceptible to infection by the human papilloma virus in contrast to its increased susceptibility to other cutaneous viral infections such as herpes zoster.

The benign melanocytic naevi have an interesting natural history.[1] Relatively few of these lesions are present at birth or develop in the first 5 years of life. Throughout childhood it is normal to develop a small number of melanocytic naevi, but the bulk of melanocytic naevi first make themselves visible around puberty. For the next 10–20 years numbers of melanocytic naevi are maximal on the body surface at approximately 20–40 naevi per individual. Thereafter there is a slow decline in visible naevi so that in old age numbers of naevi are less than 10 per individual. This interesting sequence is interpreted on the basis of pathological studies of naevi taken from all age-ranges as representing maturation and ageing of the naevi. Melanocytic naevi are initially predominantly related to the dermo-epidermal junction. In early adult life the majority of melanocytic naevi excised have naevus cells both in the dermo-epidermal junction area and lying free in the dermis, the so-called compound naevus. In later adult life the bulk of excised naevi show activity only in the dermis. It is therefore assumed that the cells comprising these naevi go through a sequence of early proliferation at the dermo-epidermal junction area, that some of these descend into the underlying dermis, but that with maturation these cells lose their ability to proliferate and the naevi disappear. From this detailed account of naevus cell biology, it will be clear that a new pigmented lesion appearing in late adult life is most unlikely to be a benign naevus and must be regarded with some suspicion.

At the present time there is great interest in the association between various types of cutaneous malignancy and sun exposure. This is an important area of geriatric dermatology as many of the clinically visible changes in the human skin that are interpreted as signs of ageing are more appropriately attributed to the results of lifetime exposure to sun and wind, a so-called weathering effect. Clinical comparison of the weathered skin of the cheek of an 80-year-old with the unexposed skin of the lower back or buttock area on the same patient will illustrate very clearly that while ageing *per se* may be associated with some dryness, laxity and perhaps loss of pigmentation, very much more striking changes are seen on the light-exposed sites in the form of wrinkling, scaling and pigmentary abnormalities. Although a high proportion of the majority of types of cutaneous malignancy are found on the habitually exposed skin of the face and back of the hand, the higher incidence of cutaneous malignancy in the elderly is seen in parts of the world in which there are long hours of natural sunlight and also in parts of the world in which there is much less natural sunlight. A small proportion of cutaneous malignancies and pre-malignant lesions are found on rarely exposed skin sites, and these too are commoner in older than in younger individuals. There is thus a complex relationship between the ageing process, exposure to ultraviolet radiation and the incidence of cutaneous malignancy. There is, however, no doubt that many of the changes traditionally associated with pre-malignancy, and in particular actinic keratoses, are found at a very much younger age in white-skinned races in parts of the world in which there are long hours of natural sunlight, notably Australia.[2]

The following conditions are discussed in this chapter:

Solar or actinic keratoses
Disseminated superficial actinic porokeratosis
Erythema ab igne
Cutaneous horn
Keratoacanthoma
Bowen's disease
Pre-malignant leucoplakia and erythroplakia of the mucous membranes
Basal cell carcinoma
Squamous cell carcinoma
Malignant melanoma

SOLAR OR ACTINIC KERATOSES (*Fig.* 9.1)

These lesions are extremely common on the face and hands of individuals over the age of 70 years in the UK, and of very much younger individuals in the sunnier parts of the world such as Australia.

No good epidemiological study comparing the incidence of actinic keratoses in various races has been carried out, and the bulk of the literature on these lesions is confined to studies of Caucasians. Personal experience would suggest that actinic keratoses are relatively rare on dark-skinned patients, suggesting that melanin pigment does afford some protection against these lesions.

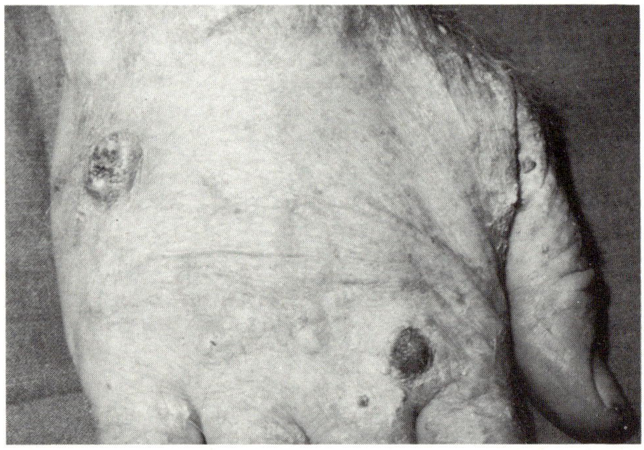

Fig. 9.1 Actinic keratosis. Note scaling warty lesions on the back of the hands of a retired farmer.

They are found mainly on the face and on the backs of the hands. The lesions are recognized clinically as rough erythematous scaling areas of skin that remain relatively static over long periods of time. On the cheek area they may be easily traumatized by shaving and give rise to bleeding.

The pathological features of actinic keratoses are the result of a loss of the normal maturation and differentiation process of the epidermal keratinocyte, which is a cell terminally differentiated and committed to produce the superficial stratum corneum of the epidermis. In actinic keratoses the orderly maturation pattern of small dark keratinocytes at the basal layer of the epidermis, maturing to flat anucleate squames at the epidermal surface, is lost. There is alternating parakeratosis and orthokeratosis, and in the dermis underlying the areas of epidermal change there may be a mild lymphocytic infiltrate. An interesting pathological feature of these lesions is the fact that the epidermis overlying the skin appendages (hair follicles and sweat glands) appears to be less affected than the intervening areas. The late Herman Pinkus has suggested that this is because the stem cells in the area of the skin appendages may receive a greater degree of protection from ultraviolet radiation than adjacent stem cells and this may explain the unusual pattern.

If untreated, a proportion of actinic keratoses may progress to frank squamous cell carcinoma. In the past, figures of 20–50 per cent have been quoted for this progression, but recent excellent work carried out in Melbourne has suggested that this may be as low as 5 per cent in Australia,[3] and that if skin is protected from ultraviolet radiation there may be a significant regression rate in these lesions. These recent observations are of great importance in view of the ageing population in the UK and the current enthusiasm for prolonged exposure of Caucasian skin to ultraviolet radiation.

Signs suggesting that squamous cell carcinoma has developed within a pre-existing keratosis include the development of induration of the lesion with a firm palpable area both beneath and to the edge of the scaling and crusted area. Persistent bleeding may also be a disturbing feature suggesting malignancy.

The management of actinic keratoses once the diagnosis is established is initially prevention of further exposure to ultraviolet radiation. Restriction of hours of exposure to sunlight, the use of a hat and the use of one of the newer, extremely effective sun-screening preparations with a sun protection factor (SPF) of 8 or higher are all recommended. After 3–6 months on this type of regimen there may be considerable regression of the keratoses. The use of keratolytic preparations such as 1–5 per cent salicylic acid in Vaseline may be of value if roughness of the skin is a significant problem but is purely a symptomatic rather than a therapeutic measure. Mild cryotherapy is of great value in the management of individual lesions and if used selectively can result in complete cure of large areas of keratoses. The use of topical cytotoxics may also be of value. Topical 5-fluorouracil (5-FU) (Efudix) has an interesting property of selectively localizing in areas of maximum epidermal disturbance. If topical 5-FU is applied to the skin it will be found that erythema develops maximally in those areas in which there is clear clinical evidence of actinic keratosis, but also in areas adjacent to these sites. Biopsy of these clinically normal areas will reveal that there is pathological evidence of actinic damage in these sites. Thus 5-FU selectively localizes in areas of both clinical and preclinical actinic damage. The preparation must be handled with care under supervision as it can damage the eyes and mucous membranes. A suitable regimen is application of topical 5-FU nightly to the affected areas for 2–3 weeks. During the last week of therapy the cutaneous lesions may temporarily look very much more inflamed, but after treatment is discontinued there will usually be a significant and worthwhile regression that may be confirmed histologically. Most studies suggest that topical 5-FU is very much more effective on facial skin than on other body sites.

Surgical excision is rarely appropriate in actinic keratoses because of the multifocal nature of the problem. At present there is considerable interest in the use, both topically and systemically, of the retinoid group of drugs. This group of drugs has chemical formulae similar to vitamin A, and a number of them have promise as possible cytostatic or cytotoxic agents. Trials of topical and systemic etretinate and 13-*cis*-retinoic acid are currently in progress and there have been reports of worthwhile remission of actinic keratosis during systemic administration.[4] Experience does, however, suggest that actinic keratoses may well recur immediately the drug is withdrawn, and troublesome side-effects may be associated with systemic use.

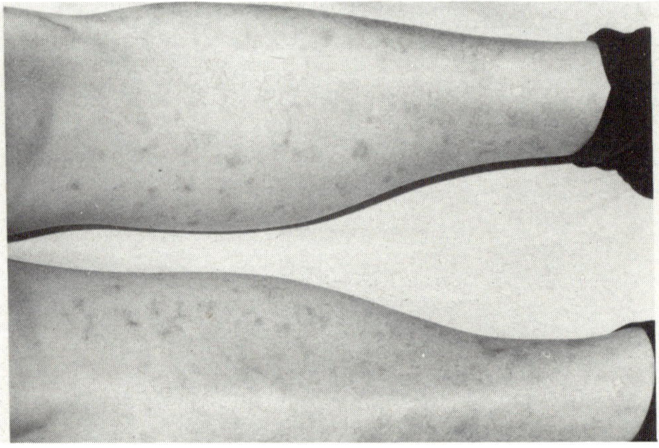

Fig. 9.2. Disseminated superficial actinic porokeratosis. Note numerous small circular lesions on the lower legs of a 70-year-old female.

DISSEMINATED SUPERFICIAL ACTINIC POROKERATOSIS (*Fig*. 9.2)

This interesting condition was first described in 1967. The clinical appearances of these lesions, which are usually multiple, are of small circular scaling lesions, usually 1 cm or less in diameter, commonly found on the lower legs particularly in older females. Careful examination with a hand lens will show that there is a raised threadlike margin to these lesions, associated with some central atrophy. Although the term 'actinic' is used in the description of these lesions, not all patients have a history of significant or excessive sun exposure.

These lesions require pathological confirmation of the clinical diagnosis. The pathological feature that is diagnostic of all porokeratotic conditions is the presence of the so-called cornoid lamella, which is seen on histological examination as a striking feather-like plume of parakeratosis surrounded by areas of normally keratinized epidermis.

The importance of porokeratosis is the fact that in a small proportion of cases there may be progression to frank squamous cell carcinoma. The interested reader is referred to a recent editorial on all types of porokeratosis.[5]

This condition can be controlled with cryotherapy with a liquid nitrogen spray. Once the condition is diagnosed these patients should be kept under regular review because of the possibility of malignant change.

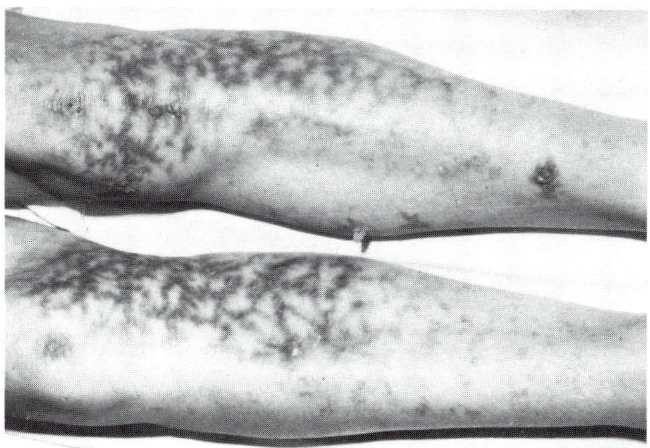

Fig. 9.3. Erythema ab igne. Note the striking mottled pattern on the calves of this elderly female who sits for much of the day over a coal fire.

ERYTHEMA AB IGNE (*Fig.* 9.3)

This condition is most commonly seen on the lower legs of elderly patients, usually female, who have no central heating and who rely on a source of radiant heat, either a coal or an electric fire, as their sole method of heating. It is relatively common in certain parts of Scotland and enjoys the popular name 'tinker's tartan'. Until recently in the United States the condition was unheard of because central heating was so commonly available. However, in the past 10 years the condition has been identified in some of the less affluent parts of the United States.

The clinical presentation of this condition is that of a mottled or marbled pattern of erythema on the lower legs, usually on the inner surface of both calves and knees. The pattern follows no recognized distribution of either nerve supply or vascular supply. If the stimulus is removed the condition is partially reversible, but if the elderly patient continues to sit close to a source of radiant heat the erythematous reticular lesions will become raised and crusted and may in time develop frank malignant change (*Fig.* 9.4).

The pathology of these lesions is very similar to that seen in the actinic keratoses described earlier.

The management of this condition is the provision of a more uniform source of heat. If the possibility of malignant change is considered, an excision biopsy of the area in question should be carried out.

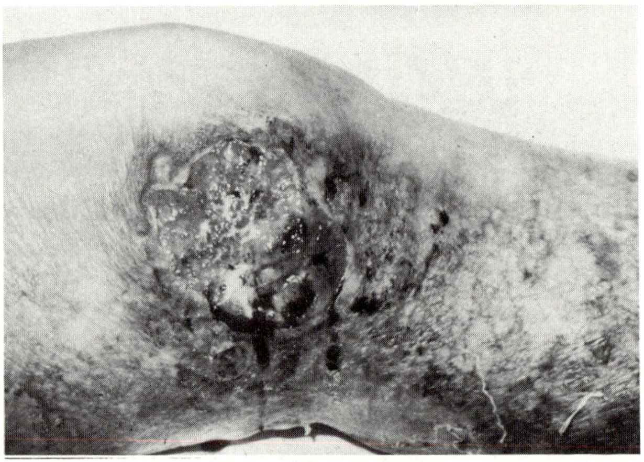

Fig. 9.4. Squamous cell carcinoma that has developed on a previous site of erythema ab igne. By the time this elderly female presented for treatment she already had secondary tumour in the lymph nodes in the groin.

CUTANEOUS HORN

This term is a purely clinical descriptive term. It is self-explanatory but the important point to bear in mind is the fact that this gross disorder of keratinization arises on the basis of an abnormal underlying epidermis. It is important to establish whether or not this underlying abnormality is merely a benign epidermal dysplasia or an early frank malignancy of the epidermis. For this reason cutaneous horns should not be treated merely by removal of the outer keratinized area but the base of the lesion should be excised and examined histologically.

KERATOACANTHOMA (*Fig.* 9.5)

This is an interesting type of cutaneous tumour that occupies an indeterminate position between benign and malignant epidermal lesions. It is found predominantly on light-exposed skin and on hair-bearing areas. This may include the face, the ears and backs of the hands. The clinical picture is that of a very rapidly growing, raised, usually spherical lesion. The lesion may appear and grow to a diameter of 3–4 cm over a period of 2–3 weeks, giving rise to great concern about rapidly developing malignancy. The classic keratoacanthoma, however, ceases growing after a period of weeks, and thereafter the central part undergoes degeneration and breaks down to form a crater. This appearance is then maintained for a further short period of time and the lesion involutes completely, usually leaving a rather disfiguring and irregular scar.

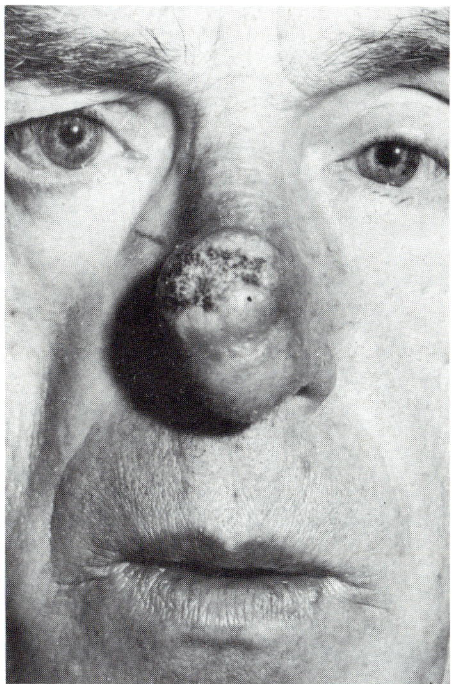

Fig. 9.5. Keratoacanthoma. Note the crusted lesion on the nose of this elderly male. This lesion has only been present for 3 weeks.

The aetiology of this rapidly growing but spontaneously regressing tumour is not understood. In the past it has been suggested that these lesions arise on the basis of hair follicles, which normally have their own inbuilt growth and resting phases. This has not yet, however, been proved. Their clinical importance lies in the fact that a small proportion of squamous cell carcinomas may clinically be very similar to keratoacanthoma.

The pathology of keratoacanthoma can only be accurately interpreted if the pathologist is given an appropriate biopsy from the lesion in question. It is essential that a full-thickness wedge of tissue is taken through the apparently deepest part of the lesion. The characteristic feature of keratoacanthoma is a striking cup-shape invagination of epidermis that forms the edge of the central crater area. This is the most useful feature for the pathologist to identify. The pathological differential diagnosis between keratoacanthoma and squamous cell carcinoma may on occasion be very difficult indeed because of the fact that the deeper part of a keratoacanthoma may contain apparently isolated nests of epidermal cells lying free in the dermis in a manner very similar to that seen in an invasive cell squamous carcinoma.

The management of keratoacanthoma may be either active or passive. If the diagnosis is clinically and pathologically obvious and the patient is elderly, it may be considered appropriate merely to observe the lesion for the natural shrinkage and allow for the fact that the residual scar may be cosmetically less than perfect. In many situations, however, it is considered more appropriate to remove the lesion either by shaving or by full excision. This will in most cases result in a cosmetically more acceptable scar, and will of course allow for full pathological examination and confirmation of the benign nature of the lesion. If the passive and expectant approach to treatment is adopted it is recommended that this be permitted only for lesions that have been present for less than 4 months. It is the author's opinion that lesions present for longer than this may well be slow growing, well-differentiated squamous cell carcinomas and therefore should be excised.

BOWEN'S DISEASE (INTRAEPIDERMAL CARCINOMA *IN SITU*) (*Fig.* 9.6)

This interesting condition is one of two types of malignancy that appear to be confined in the vast majority of cases to the epidermis. There is thus proliferation of cells that have cytological features strongly suggestive of frank malignant change, but metastasis very rarely, if ever, occurs.

The clinical feature of Bowen's disease is the presence, usually on covered sites of the body, of an isolated scaling erythematous patch. This patch may grow over a period of months to a size of several centimetres in diameter. It is not uncommon for this lesion to be diagnosed initially as an isolated patch of psoriasis, and referral for specialist opinion to take place only when conventional antipsoriatic treatment fails to clear the lesion. If left untreated the majority of these lesions will slowly expand and involve greater areas of the epidermal surface. A very small proportion of cases of Bowen's disease have been reported in which metastasis beyond the epidermis has taken place.

In the past patients who have been given arsenical preparations in tonic in childhood have been reported as having a higher incidence of Bowen's disease in old age.

The pathological features of Bowen's disease are the presence within the epidermis of gross epidermal dysplasia with very large epidermal cells exhibiting atypical mitoses and premature keratinization. One recent study has suggested that a type of human papilloma virus may be seen in cases of Bowen's disease.

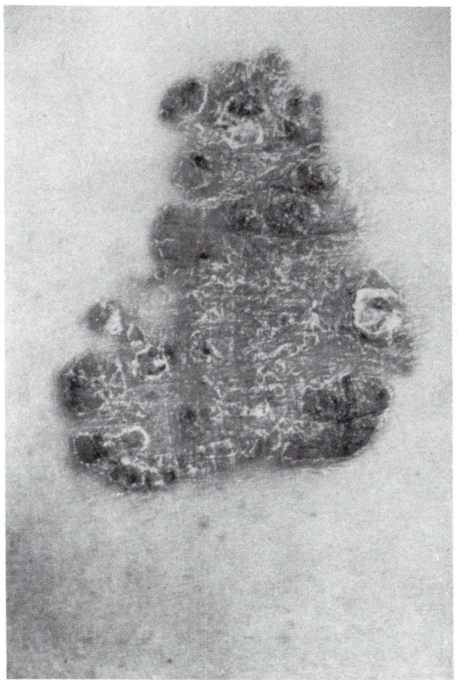

Fig. 9.6. Bowen's disease. Scaling isolated lesion on the lower back of a 73-year-old female.

The management of Bowen's disease once the diagnosis is pathologically confirmed by biopsy may either be by excision or by radiotherapy as this lesion is radiosensitive. Other less aggressive measures such as cryotherapy are not usually effective in totally eradicating the lesions and should not be undertaken in patients unless they are very elderly and frail.

PRE-MALIGNANT LEUCOPLAKIA AND ERYTHROPLAKIA OF THE MUCOUS MEMBRANES

Oral mucosal lesions in the elderly may also be pre-malignant. In the past there has been some confusion over the term 'leucoplakia' (literally white patches) in that it was considered that these lesions were pre-malignant. White patches on the oral mucous membrane of elderly patients are very common indeed and may be due either to simple atrophy of the mucous membrane, or to mild chronic candidosis due to dentures being colonized with *Candida albicans*. This is not a pre-malignant problem, but the elderly patient with white patches alternating with areas of inflammation—leucoerythroplakia—is at risk of malignant change. This problem is seen more commonly in smokers and in those with poor dental hygiene. Any persisting red velvety raised area on the oral mucous membranes should be biopsied to exclude oral carcinoma.

BASAL CELL CARCINOMA

This is the commonest type of skin tumour at any age, and is the second of the group of intra-epidermal malignancies that very rarely metastasize. It is not yet established whether or not these common tumours do indeed arise from the basal cells of the epidermis or possibly from a portion of the hair follicle epithelium.

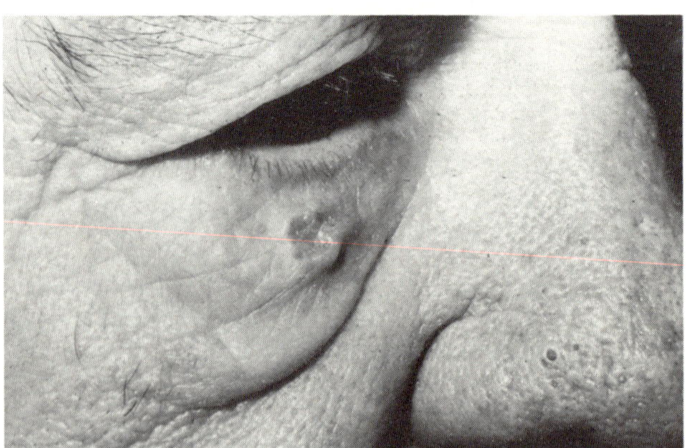

Fig. 9.7. Classic basal cell carcinoma. Note the raised, curly edge with incipient ulceration below the right eye.

The clinical features of basal cell carcinoma may vary considerably. The classic lesion or rodent ulcer is a raised, rather translucent papule that grows slowly, most commonly on the face and in particular in the inner canthus area (*Fig*. 9.7). This lesion may expand over a period of

1–2 years and then develop a central ulcerated area. If this lesion is not treated it may grow relentlessly and destroy bone, cartilage and other tissue. The destructive results of large basal cell carcinomas are not sometimes fully appreciated (*Fig.* 9.8), and it is important to realize that local invasion may cause results just as devastating as distant metastases.

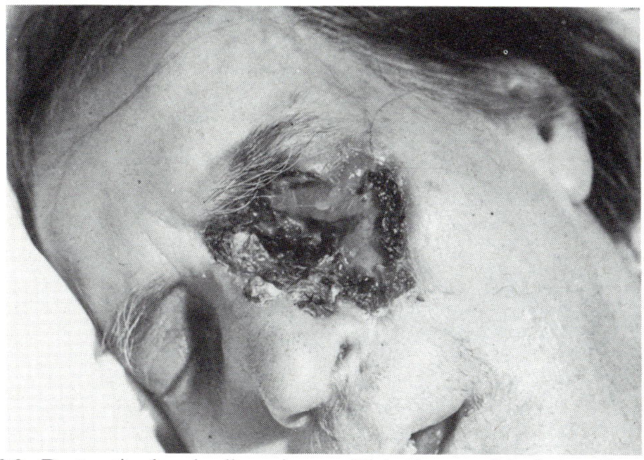

Fig. 9.8. Destructive basal cell carcinoma. Note the complete destruction of the orbital area in this elderly female. Note the raised pearly border seen at the margin of the lesion.

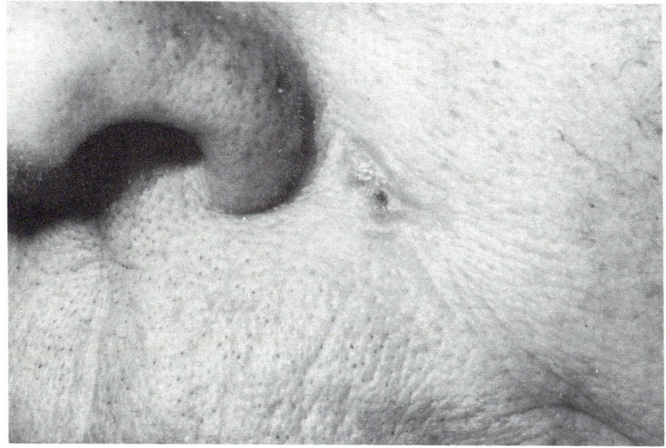

Fig. 9.9. Morphoeic basal cell carcinoma. Note the small crusted scar-like area adjacent to the nostril.

A troublesome variant of basal cell carcinoma is the morphoeic type, which develops most commonly around the nasal folds (*Fig.* 9.9).

These lesions have a clinically different presentation in that they may appear like a small scar in a site in which there is no past history of trauma. It is particularly important to ensure that this type of tumour is completely excised as it may extend surprisingly deeply along tissue planes, and local recurrence is extremely common.

Extrafacial basal cell carcinomas are much less common than those found on the face, but may be confusing clinically (*Fig*. 9.10). The most common problem is differentiation from Bowen's disease. A helpful clinical feature is the presence of a raised, slightly rolled margin to the lesion in the case of the basal cell carcinomas. This feature is absent in Bowen's disease. If there is any clinical doubt, biopsy will confirm the nature of the lesion.

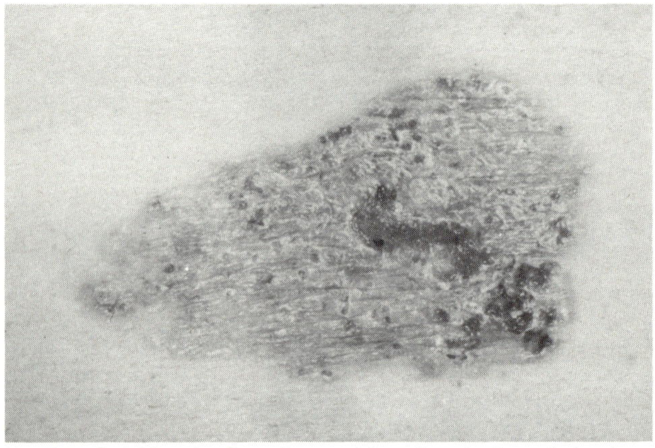

Fig. 9.10. Extrafacial basal cell carcinoma. Note the raised pearly border at the lower margin of the lesion.

A rare familial problem is that of Gorlin's syndrome or the multiple basal cell naevus syndrome. This is transmitted by autosomal dominant inheritance, and the unfortunate patients develop very large numbers of basal cell carcinomas in early adult life. The importance of recognizing this syndrome lies in the fact that while the classic basal cell carcinoma may quite reasonably be treated by radiotherapy (*see below*), patients with Gorlin's syndrome may well develop multiple new tumours in the irradiated field and excision is therefore more appropriate treatment.

Basal cell carcinoma may develop in two types of congenital epidermal abnormalities. These are the organoid or sebaceous naevus, and the naevus syringocystadenoma papilliferum. In both situations the basal cell carcinomas tend to develop relatively early in life, and neither is likely to be a problem in the geriatric field.

The pathological feature of basal cell carcinoma is the presence of tongues of epidermal cells invading downwards into the underlying dermis but still retaining contact with the epidermis. These apparently invasive areas are demarcated by a clear pallisade of small, darkly staining basal cells beyond which there is a stroma that is part of the tumour. These features are characteristic and the condition is usually easily confirmed on biopsy.

The treatment of basal cell carcinoma may be either by surgical excision or by radiotherapy. The patient's condition and local facilities will determine which is more appropriate. Less definitive therapeutic measures such as cryotherapy are not recommended as definitive treatment, and should be reserved for local control of disease in patients who are very frail.

SQUAMOUS CELL CARCINOMA

Squamous cell carcinoma is seen most commonly on 'weathered' skin, usually the face and hands (*Fig.* 9.11). There may be a past history of actinic keratoses. Other predisposing factors include erythema ab igne (*see* p. 113), sites of chronic skin trauma such as ulcers or burns or scars on the site of previously treated lupus vulgaris. Certain chemical carcinogens in tars, soot and cutting oils may also predispose to squamous cell carcinoma. The classic historical example of this is the scrotal squamous cell carcinoma first described in chimney sweeps by Percival Potts.

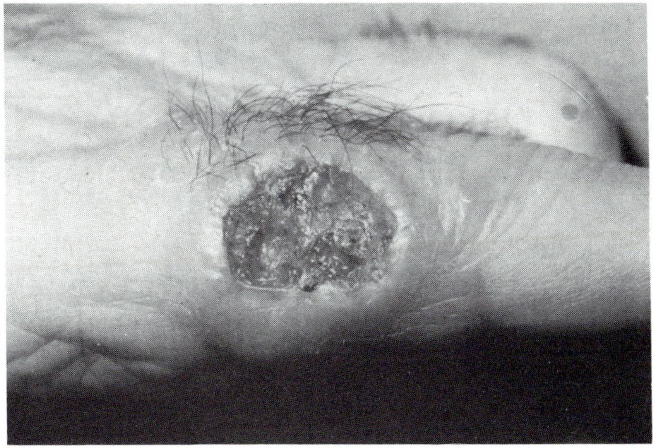

Fig. 9.11. Squamous cell carcinoma on the side of the hand developing in a patient with multiple previous actinic keratoses.

There is also recent evidence that immunosuppression may predispose to squamous cell carcinoma, particularly in association with sunlight exposure.[6,7] This evidence comes from studies of renal transplant patients who have a much higher than expected incidence of non-Hodgkin's lymphoma and also of non-melanoma skin cancer. There is as yet no clear evidence of a similar problem in patients on long-term immunosuppressants for connective tissue disease or other similar conditions.

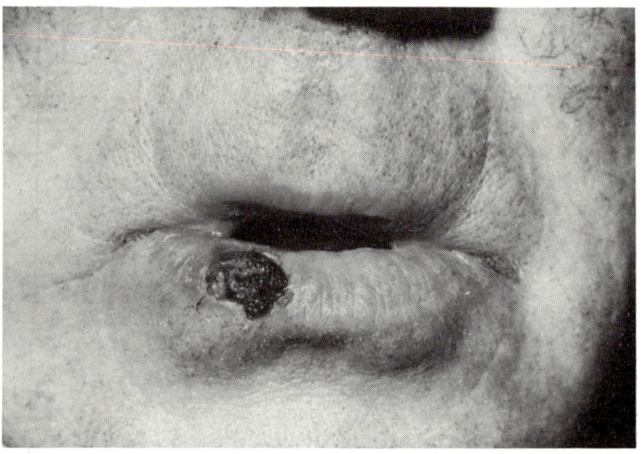

Fig. 9.12. Squamous cell carcinoma of the lower lip in an elderly male. Note the fullness along the lip, indicating that there are multiple areas of malignant cells in this site.

The clinical presentation of squamous cell carcinoma is that of an expanding, usually ulcerated nodule on the skin surface. These lesions may metastasize relatively early to the lymph nodes, and there is some evidence to suggest that tumours arising on the lip (*Fig.* 9.12) and on scarred areas do so earlier than those arising on actinic keratoses. The possibility of squamous cell carcinoma developing on a longstanding ulcerated area, particularly a leg ulcer, should be considered if a firm, raised nodule develops, usually at the edge of the ulcer.

The diagnostic pathological feature of squamous cell carcinoma is the presence in the dermis of isolated groups of malignant cells derived from the overlying epidermis. These groups of cells may show varying degrees of inappropriate keratinization.

The treatment of squamous cell carcinoma may be by either surgery or radiotherapy. In general, bearing in mind the fact that squamous cell carcinoma commonly develops on skin already damaged by ultraviolet radiation or other factors, it is more logical to use surgical excision provided the patient's condition and local facilities allow.

Radiotherapy has a useful part to play in palliation and in some cases in the cure of squamous cell carcinoma but in general is perhaps a second choice of treatment.

MALIGNANT MELANOMA

The incidence of malignant melanoma is rising steadily in all countries in the world for which accurate incidence figures are available. Age-adjusted incidence rates show that the incidence rises sharply in those over the age of 60. The condition is very much commoner in white-skinned races, the ratio of white to black patients affected in areas where both lead a similar lifestyle being 10:1. In the UK twice as many females are affected as males.

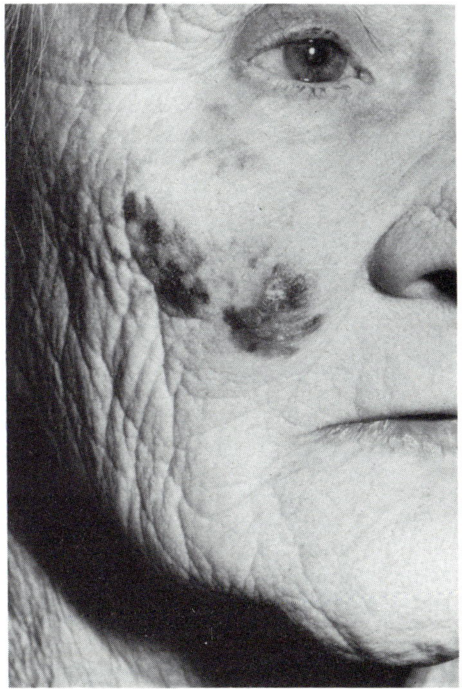

Fig. 9.13. Lentigo maligna melanoma in the cheek of an 80-year-old. A brown macular area had been present in the cheek for 8 years previously.

Malignant melanoma can be divided on clinicopathological grounds into four main types: (1) superficial spreading malignant melanoma, which comprises approximately half of all cases in Europe and North America; (2) nodular melanoma, which comprises approximately 20 per cent of cases; (3) lentigo maligna melanoma, which comprises 15 per cent of all cases; and (4) acral lentiginous melanoma, which comprises the remaining 15 per cent. In the elderly it is the lentigo maligna melanoma and the acral lentiginous type that are most likely to present and give rise to problems.

The lentigo maligna melanoma arises mainly on the face, most commonly on the cheek (*Fig*. 9.13). The clinical presentation here is that the patient will give a history of having had a macular brown area on the skin surface present for may years. Family photographs may confirm the presence of such a lesion 5 or 10 years previously. The lesion may slowly expand across the skin of the cheek and may indeed undergo central regression. After a very variable period of time, however, a central raised roughened or nodular area may develop. This is an indication that the lesion has passed from the intra-epidermal or radial growth phase, which may be called Hutchinson's pre-malignant freckle, precancerous melanosis of Dubreulh or lentigo maligna. The lesion is now an invasive malignant melanoma.

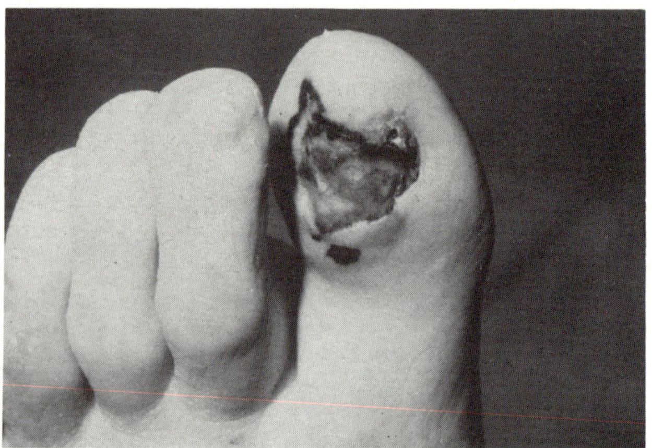

Fig. 9.14. Periungual malignant melanoma of the toe. This patient had been receiving treatment from a chiropodist until 1 week before the photograph was taken.

The acral or acral lentiginous melanoma is found most commonly on the soles of the feet and particularly in the periungual area (*Fig*. 9.14). The ratio of these lesions on the feet to the hands in a large Scottish series was 8:1.[8] These lesions present as slowly expanding macular brown lesions on the skin of the foot, which in time develop raised nodular areas. The malignant melanomas that develop around the nail may be difficult to recognize in the early stages and for this reason may be inappropriately treated as ingrowing toenails or warts before the true nature of the condition is recognized. It is extremely important that chiropodists, district nurses and others involved in the care of the elderly, and in particular in the care of their feet, are aware of the clinical features that may suggest early periungual melanoma. Most of these lesions do show some pigmentation. In many situations this may be confused with a simple bruise under the nail arising because of trauma. A very important sign in this situation is the presence of brown pigmentation on the skin of the nailfold immediately proximal to the nail. This pigmentation, called Hutchinson's sign, is a very important indication that the pigment under the nail itself is likely to be melanin associated with malignant melanoma rather than altered blood following haemorrhage. If there is any doubt whatever about the nature of a pigmented lesion on the nailbed the nail should be removed and the nailbed subjected to biopsy.

The pathological feature of malignant melanoma is the presence of malignant melanocytes invading the dermis. In the normal situation melanocytes are found only in the basal layer of the epidermis. In older patients the numbers of melanocytes in normal skin fall slightly, although larger numbers are seen on habitually sun-exposed skin. Thus melanocyte counts on the outer aspect of the upper arm are higher than those on the inner aspect in elderly patients.

Malignant melanoma is a tumour that may metastasize both to regional lymph nodes and to distant sites and thus be fatal. The prognosis for the individual patient with malignant melanoma can be gauged relatively accurately nowadays by measuring the Bresslow or tumour thickness of the primary lesion. This is done quite simply by measuring in millimetres, using an ocular micrometre in the microscope, the distance from the granular layers of the epidermis to the deepest invasive melanoma cell in the dermis. Melanomas that are less than 1·5 mm thick by this technique have a very good 5-year survival rate with over 90 per cent of patients surviving tumour free. In contrast patients with tumours 3 mm or greater in thickness have a 5-year survival rate of less than 40 per cent.

The treatment of malignant melanoma is by surgical excision. The extent of this excision is a matter of some debate. In the case of lesions on the face removal of the entire pigmented area with a 1-cm margin of normal skin is ideal but may not be feasible because of proximity to the ocular area. In the case of periungual lesions on the feet, amputation of the digit is often the most appropriate measure. Malignant melanoma may metastasize to draining lymph nodes and these patients should be reviewed at regular intervals. If nodes become clinically palpable a full node dissection should be carried out. At present there is no proven effective chemotherapy for melanoma used in either a therapeutic or an adjuvant setting.

OTHER RARE TYPES OF SKIN TUMOUR

There is a wide range of skin tumours that arise from the skin appendages. These may be related to the sweat glands, the sebaceous glands and the hair follicles. In general these lesions present as raised lumps on the skin and have no specific diagnostic clinical features. Pathological examination is essential to make a diagnosis. In the great majority of cases these lesions behave in a manner similar to basal cell carcinoma in that they may grow and recur locally but rarely metastasize.

CUTANEOUS LYMPHOMA

Cutaneous lymphomas are seen more commonly on the elderly than in younger individuals. The commonest type of cutaneous lymphoma, mycosis fungoides, is a malignant proliferation of T lymphocytes. Patients with this condition present with itchy erythematous plaques on the trunk and limbs.

Biopsy of these lesions will show the presence of atypical T lymphocytes in both the epidermis and the underlying dermis. This condition may be confined to the skin for many years with no evidence of involvement of lymph nodes or other organs.

The management of cutaneous lymphoma is best carried out in the elderly on a symptomatic basis. It is relatively easy to control the discomfort and pruritus of mycosis fungoides, but difficult to eradicate the condition completely. The itch arising from the condition can be controlled with photochemotherapy (PUVA), with superficial X-ray therapy or with topical applications of a cytotoxic such as nitrogen mustard. All of these treatments will give good symptomatic relief and the choice of the most appropriate will depend on local availability. Systemic chemotherapy is of surprisingly little value in this condition and may in fact make the situation worse by depressing the patient's innate immunity and allowing opportunistic infection to develop.

It can be seen that the range of cutaneous malignancies and also of pre-malignant conditions that may present in the elderly is wide. With the increasing number of elderly patients in the population and the increasing enthusiasm for exposure to sunlight it is likely that in future all geriatricians and family doctors will see many more examples of all types of cutaneous malignancy. In the great majority of cases early diagnosis and prompt therapy will result in cure. It is therefore of great importance that all those involved in the care of the elderly are aware of the early clinical presentation of cutaneous malignancy.

REFERENCES

1. MacKie R. M., English J., Aitchison T.C. et al. (1985) *Br. J. Dermatol.* **113**, 167.
2. Marks R. and Selwood T. S. (1985) *Cancer* **56**, 2332.
3. Marks R. (1985) *Eur. J. Epidemiol.* **1**, 319.
4. Beretti B., Grupper C., Edelson Y. et al. (1981) In: Orfanos C. E. (ed.) *Retinoids.* Berlin, Springer-Verlag, p. 397.
5. Chernovsky M. E. (1986) *Arch. Dermatol.* **112**, 869.
6. Penn I. (1984) *Transplant. Proc.* **16**, 492.
7. Sheil A. G. R., Flavel S., Disney A. P. S. et al. (1985) *Transplant. Proc.* **17**, 1685.
8. MacKie R. M., Soutar D. S., Smyth J.F. et al. (1985) *Lancet* **ii**, 859.

10. MODERN DRESSINGS FOR LEG ULCERS

M. Varghese and D. M. Carter

Ulceration of the legs is not an uncommon medical problem and has been observed more frequently in older individuals. This may be caused by a wide variety of both systemic and local disease processes (*Table* 10.1).[1,2] Local vascular disturbance remains the most common factor in the development of these ulcers, and venous insufficiency accounts for more than two-thirds of all cases. Prompt attention to aetiological factors and local supportive and topical care of these ulcers often lead to complete healing. However, due to inability to eliminate the causative factors or due to some unknown reason, a few of these ulcers fail to heal and remain chronic. Persistent infection, obesity and ageing all compound the problem. These chronic ulcers incur significant morbidity in afflicted individuals in addition to the time and cost required for their management. Favourable modulation of local wound environment may enhance healing of chronic ulcers. Biosynthetic dressings, considered later in this chapter, are sometimes effective in this regard.[3]

Until two to three decades ago it was commonly held that the formation of a dry scab is beneficial for wound healing. However, in 1962 Winter[4] showed that epithelialization is retarded by dry eschar and if eschar formation can be prevented the rate of epithelialization can be markedly increased. In his study using domestic pigs, he demonstrated that the rate of epithelialization is clearly faster in wounds kept moist by polyethylene film in comparison with wounds left exposed to air. Normal eschar on a wound exposed to air includes the superficial part of dermis that is dry and impedes epidermal migration. Impairment in epithelialization is exaggerated if the wound is kept dry artificially at 40 °C.[5] Hinman and Maibach[6] demonstrated similar, more rapid re-epithelialization in human experimental split-thickness wounds occluded with polyethylene film than in air-exposed controls. In evaluating the effect of local wound environment on epidermal healing Rovee et al.[7] found a decrease in the magnitude and duration of mitotic response in occluded wounds as opposed to air-exposed wounds. The time of onset of mitosis after wounding was comparable. The decrease in mitotic response was accompanied by a

Table 10.1. Causes of leg ulcers

A. Vascular Diseases	
1. Arterial	2. Venous
Thromboangitis obliterans	Venous stasis
Arteriosclerosis obliterans	3. Lymphatic
Hypertensive ulcer	Elephantiasis nostra
Chilblains	Lymphoedema
B. Vasculitides	
Rheumatoid arthritis	Necrotizing angiitis
Lupus erythematosus	Cryoglobulinaemia
Scleroderma	Allergic vasculitis
Periarteritis nodosa	Livedoid vasculitis
C. Metabolic Disorders	
Diabetes mellitus	Porphyria cutanea tarda
Necrobiosis lipoidica	Gaucher's disease
Gout	
D. Haematological Diseases	
Sickle cell anaemia	Leukaemia
Thalassaemia	Dysproteinaemia
Polycythaemia vera	
E. Drugs	
Halogens	Erogotism
Bromide	Methotrexate
Iodide	
F. Infection	
1. Bacterial	4. Fungal
2. Spirochaetal	Blastomycosis
3. Mycobacteria	Sporotricosis
Tuberculosis	Cryptococcus
Leprosy	Coccidioidomycosis
Atypical mycobacteria	Histoplasmosis
	Maduromycosis
	5. Protozoan
G. Malignant Tumours	
Basal cell carcinoma	Lymphoma
Squamous cell carcinoma	Mycosis fungoides
Malignant melanoma	Lymphosarcoma
Kaposi's sarcoma	Metastatic carcinoma
H. Miscellaneous	
Pyoderma gangrenosum	Radiation
Trauma	Panniculitis
Pressure Sores	Lichen planus
Burns	Factitial
Chemical	Trophic ulcers
Thermal	

shortened duration for re-epithelialization and stratification. They concluded that re-epithelialization is primarily dependent on epidermal cell migration, and that migration is independent of mitosis in the healing process.

The importance of oxygen as an essential component in the healing process has been demonstrated in the past. Various investigators have reported that increasing the partial pressure of oxygen locally can increase the rate of epithelialization and collagen production.[8,9,10] More resurfacing was noted with occluded wounds covered by polypropylene film, which had 60 times more oxygen permeability than wounds covered with polyester film, with low oxygen permeability.[8] Further acceleration of epithelialization could be demonstrated with hyperbaric oxygen. Collagen synthesis was also increased above normal with an increase in local tissue oxygen tension and was roughly proportional to arterial oxygen tension.[10] In an infected wound the oxygen tension rapidly dropped to zero and remained so for a prolonged period.[11] This was accompanied by a significant decrease in collagen synthesis. Information such as this led to the concept that ambient oxygen tension, similar in amount to that of atmospheric oxygen, might be necessary for the rapid healing of wounds. Synthetic wound dressings were developed composed of semi-permeable transparent membranes, which allow oxygen and moisture to pass through but exclude bacteria. Advances in cell biology and biochemistry in recent years have further enhanced our knowledge of wound healing. It is now known that reduced partial pressure of oxygen promotes *in vitro* growth of fibroblasts and production of angiogenesis factor from tissue macrophages.[12,13] In experiments on domestic pigs, comparing oxygen-impermeable hydrocolloid dressings, oxygen-permeable polyurethane film and wet-to-dry gauze, Alvarez et al.[14] have demonstrated an increased rate of re-epithelialization with both oxygen-permeable and impermeable dressings. Relative collagen production was also increased under both these dressings compared to wet-to-dry gauze and air-exposed wounds. Studies like these seriously challenged the notion that increased ambient oxygen tension is beneficial in wound healing.

One disadvantage of occlusive dressings is the possibility that infection may develop.[15] Quantitative bacteriological evaluation of skin under Vinylidene polymer plastic film showed an increase in *Staphylococcus aureus* in atopic skin.[16] However, bacteriological evaluations with some of the newer synthetic dressings have produced contrary results. Mertz et al.,[17] for example, found that some of these dressings provide protective barrier properties to wounds from invasion by pathogenic bacteria. In our own laboratories we have also demonstrated that the local pH of the wound is influenced by some of these dressings, which may affect bacterial growth.[18] We found that the pH of the wound fluid under a hydrocolloid dressing was approximately 6·0. The decrease in pH had an inhibitory effect on the growth of three bacteria: *Staphylococcus aureus*, *Escherichia coli* and *Pseudomonas aeruginosa*, commonly isolated from chronic ulcers.

SYNTHETIC WOUND COVERINGS

Several synthetic wound coverings and skin substitutes have been developed to promote the process of wound healing.[2,3,19,20] Some dressings in current use are listed in *Table* 10.2. By definition, wound dressings are materials designed to be replaced at regular intervals. Skin substitutes, on the other hand, are either biological wound coverings or synthetic or composite material.[20] Some of these wound coverings have been evaluated and used in the healing of leg ulcers. They vary in their properties and mechanisms of action. In common,

Table 10.2. Modern dressings/treatments for leg ulcers

Synthetic

1. Semi-permeable polyurethane films:
   OpSite, Bioclusive, Tegaderm, Polyskin, Ensure
2. Hydrogel dressings:
   Vigilon, Second Skin, Scherisorb, Geliperm, Epi-Lock, Synthaderm
3. Hydrocolloid dressings:
   DuoDERM, Granuflex, Verihesive, Stomahesive, Comfeel
4. Absorption dressings
   a. Dextranomer beads
   b. Dry polysaccharide derivative (Bard)
5. Non-adherent micropore dressing:
   Telfa, Release, Exudry, N-Terface
6. Zinc oxide paste, petroleum or Vaseline-impregnated gauze dressings:
   Unna Boot, Adaptic, Xeroform
7. Skin substitutes
   a. Bilaminate silicone membrane: Biobrane
   b. Unilaminate adherent barrier dressing: Hydron

Biological

1. Tissue derivative
   a. Collagen sheet or sponge
   b. Bioplast fibrin
2. Graft
   a. Autograft
      i. Fresh
      ii. Cultured cells
   b. Allograft
      i. Cadaveric
      ii. Amniotic membrane
   c. Xenograft (heterograft)

they provide an occlusive or semi-occlusive environment for the wound bed, preventing the wound from desiccation. They also provide a barrier to bacteria and some of them are capable of permeation by oxygen and water vapour.

Advantages of an occlusive dressing include rapid healing, reduced pain, fewer dressing changes, exclusion of micro-organisms and better cosmetic results. Main disadvantages are infection, trauma to adjacent skin, accumulation of exudate and need for healthy borders for attachment of the dressing.

Polyurethane Films

Polyvinyl chloride films, those which are commonly used for food wraps, were the first occlusive dressings tried on wounds. Their disadvantages included maceration of skin and adherence to the wound bed. Semi-permeable polyurethane films (OpSite) were first developed in England in the late 1960s to overcome these disadvantages. These films are impermeable to bacteria and water but selectively permeable to oxygen and water vapour and do not adhere to the wound bed. They have an adhesive surface at the edge for attachment to normal skin. Such materials were originally used on postoperative wounds and as surgical drapes. After several years of research and clinical application, they are now used in various clinical settings, including leg ulcers, burns and dressings for graft donor sites.

Alper et al.[21] studied 18 patients with 26 leg ulcers treated with vapour-permeable membrane (OpSite). Rapid healing was noted in all except 2; the rate of healing was reported as 2·6 times faster than in controls. Braverman and Nasar [22] evaluated OpSite in the treatment of decubitus ulcers in the elderly. Of 12 patients treated, 10 healed after 4 weeks, but only 5 subjects in the control group had healed after 4 weeks. Similar enhanced healing was noted by Avakoff.[23] Vapour-permeable membranes (OpSite) were also used successfully in treating the ulcers of osteomyelitis by Angermeier et al.[24] Two patients, with chronic ulcerations on the foot and great toe with concomitant osteomyelitis, showed complete healing and decrease in size in 2–4 months' follow-up. James and Watson[25] have used this dressing in split-thickness skin graft donor sites in 53 patients and noted the advantages of early healing, freedom from pain and lack of bulky dressings. The vapour-permeable membrane dressing has also been evaluated in burn patients by several investigators. Caldwell et al.[26] noted a decrease in evaporative water loss and heat loss with a corresponding decrease in heat production. Neal and co-workers[27] found a significantly faster healing rate in their study on burn patients.

Several variants of this dressing are available, and they vary slightly in vapour permeability, strength, flexibility and delivery systems.

OpSite has an ether-based adhesive system, whereas all others have an acrylic adhesive.[19] They have a remarkable ability to reduce pain and are non-toxic and non-sensitizing. The main disadvantages are occasional adherence to granulating wound bed and injury to newly formed epithelium at dressing change, non-adherence to normal skin at the wound edge, and the need for frequent drainage of collected material under the dressing in an exudative wound. Though considered freely permeable to oxygen, we noted marked reduction in the oxygen permeability of one of these dressings in clinical use.[18]

Hydrogel Dressings

These dressings are inert hydrogels, consisting of 4 per cent polyethylene oxide and 96 per cent water. Wichterle and Lim were the first to propose hydrogels for wound care because of the hydrophilic nature of the polymers.[28] By varying the nature of the polymer backbone, a range of water-binding behaviours and permeability properties can be achieved. Vigilon is a colloid in gelatinous sheet form consisting of an insoluble cross-linked polyethylene oxide copolymer with water as the dispersion medium. The tensile strength of this polymer is low and it is covered by a thin polyethylene film over each surface of the gel. It allows free transfer of oxygen even with an intact polyethylene film, but vapour transmission occurs at a moderate rate only with the membrane removed. Evaporation from the gel surface can be controlled by retaining the outer polyethylene film. It has a capacity to absorb wound exudate approximately to its own weight. Geronemus and Robins[29] studied its effect in partial-thickness wounds in swine and found that, in 4 days, 100 per cent of the wounds treated with this dressing healed as opposed to 32 per cent of untreated wounds. Mandy[30] evaluated its ability in accelerating the wound healing process in 26 transplantations, 42 excisional surgeries and 10 dermabrasions. All surgical excision sites appeared re-epithelialized in 48 hours and without wound infection. At 2 weeks both donor and recipient sites of hair transplantation seemed to heal faster than those of patients in the author's prior experience. Following dermabrasion, patients treated with hydrogel dressing were re-epithelialized in 4–5 days in comparison with 6–7 days in controls.

Several variants of hydrogels are available.[28] Scherisorb is a highly absorbent graft T starch polymer containing water as the dispersion medium and is comparable in structure to Vigilon. Geliperm is an insoluble, cross-linked, polyacrylamide polymer with 95 per cent water as the dispersion medium. It is also comparable to Vigilon in its properties except for a significantly reduced tensile strength, fluid absorption capacity and an increase in water vapour permeability. These hydrogel dressings are recommended as an occlusive dressing for the treatment of split-thickness wounds, burns and mild dermatoses. In chronic ulcers they are used to enhance granulation tissue. These hydrogels may promote growth of micro-organisms, especially in the presence of absorbed wound exudate, and are considered contra-indicated in necrotizing ulcerations where anaerobic infection in suspected or in deep fissure wounds or third-degree burns prior to the removal of necrotic tissue.[28]

Hydrocolloid Dressings

Hydrocolloid dressings (DuoDERM, Comfeel, Verihesive, Stomahesive, Granuflex) are occlusive dressings composed of gelatin, pectin, carboxymethyl cellulose and polyisobutylene with an outer impermeable polyurethane foam.[28] They physically interact with moisture or wound exudate, forming a hydrated gel that conforms to the wound contours and ulcer floors. They are flexible and adhesive are are impermeable to gas and moisture. They remove toxic compound but also release degradation products from the dressing into the wound that may affect the local wound environment. This type of dressing has been widely studied in the management of ulcers. Tracy et al.[31] studied 43 indolent leg ulcers treated by the application of Verihesive dressings, and 84 per cent showed healing in a mean time of 10 weeks. Similar improved rates of healing were observed by various other investigators.[32–35] Alvarez et al.[14] found an increased rate of collagen synthesis and re-epithelialization in experimental partial-thickness wounds covered with hydrocolloid dressing (DuoDERM). These dressings were also found to prevent bacterial invasion and wound infections.[16] We studied the local wound environment under these dressings and found that the pH of the wound fluid was approximately 6·0, which might induce an inhibitory effect on bacterial growth.[18] Wound angiogenesis was also increased, owing to the low oxygen concentration attained under the dressing.[36] Clinically, rapid relief of pain was noted with their usage, and they are non-sensitizing to the skin, and non-adherent to wound beds. They are easy to use and economical. The main disadvantages noted are adherence of the dressing material to the normal skin at the wound edge, making it difficult to remove, and occasional back pressure from collected exudate under the dressing onto the wound bed.

Absorption Dressings

Dextranomer, a dextran polymer, is highly hydrophilic and is manufactured in the form of dry spherical beads of 0·1–0·3 mm in diameter. This, when placed on exudative wounds, promptly absorbs serous and purulent exudate from the surface of the wound, with adherence of bacteria and other debris. The mediators of inflammation are also absorbed. Controlled animal studies have shown no difference in the rate of re-epithelialization with its use,[37] but it may aid in cleaning highly exudative and necrotic wounds and thereby facilitate healing.[38,39] Its disadvantages include dehydration of the ulcer bed, pain and haemorrhage. No allergic, irritant or toxic reaction from its use has been encountered.

Another absorption dressing (Bard) is a dry polysaccharide derivative made by graft polymerization of carboxyl and carboxamide groups onto corn starch. Its particle size ranges from 0·2–0·4 mm in diameter. When partially hydrated it forms a mouldable hydrogel and has a high absorptive capacity for water-soluble material and blood. It provides a moist physiological environment for the formation of granulation tissue, keeps tissue pliant, and minimizes eschar formation.

SKIN SUBSTITUTES

Silicone Membrane

Biobrane[40] is a bilaminate, adherent, biosynthetic skin substitute that consists of laminates of an ultra-thin, semi-permeable, silicone membrane that is mechanically bonded to a flexible, knitted nylon fabric, which is then cross-linked with porcine collagen. It is non-toxic and semi-permeable to water vapour. It adheres occlusively to wound surface and absorbs exudate, controls bacterial proliferation, reduces wound contraction and promotes re-epithelialization. It is also noted to reduce pain. Because of its flexibility, it can be used to cover irregularly contoured surfaces and joints. This has been effective in treating superficial dermal wounds and partial-thickness burns, and has been recommended for clean superficial wounds.[40,41] Its use in leg ulcers has not been evaluated.

Adherent Barrier Dressing

Polyhydroxyethyl methacrylate (Hydron) wound dressing is a unilaminate, adherent, barrier dressing for use on surfaces where the skin barrier has been compromised.[42] This is applied by mixing the polymer with a solvent polyethylene glycol. This dressing has been mainly evaluated for burn wounds. In an animal study by Nathan et al.[43] it was found to be more effective in controlling infection in surgical wounds than in burn wounds. They found a significant reduction in wound bacterial count, especially *Pseudomonas*. Only limited experience is available with this dressing, but it may be potentially useful in chronic leg ulcers.

BIOLOGICAL WOUND DRESSINGS

Grafts

Human amniotic membrane has been used as a biological wound dressing at least since 1910. Recently its role in the management of chronic leg ulcers has been re-evaluated.[44–47] Chronic ulcers of post-phlebitic, post-irradiation and post-burn origin respond to treatment more effectively with amnion dressing than do control wounds.[44] Early development of healthy granulation and development of more numerous thin-walled vessels and promotion of re-epithelialization were noted after its use. Clinically, this was associated with rapid reduction in pain and reduction in the number of bacteria in the wound. The main disadvantages of this dressing are its antigenicity and the fact it is not readily available. However, prior experience indicates that human amniotic membrane dressing can be used as an alternative biological dressing for chronic leg ulcers.[44–47]

Porcine xenografts are also used as biological dressings and have been used in burn wounds, split-thickness graft donor site, and in the preparation for autografting.[48,49] They are found to promote re-epithelialization in clean superficial wounds. Porcine heterograft can be considered a temporary biological wound dressing and is readily available commercially.

Cultured Autologous Cell Graft

Cultured autologous epidermal cell grafts have been used as a biological wound covering.[50] A small piece of epithelial tissue is grown in tissue culture to expand to a large sheet, and this has been used to cover burn wounds where the usual fresh autologous skin grafting is impossible because of extensive involvement.[51] This has also been used successfully in treating extensive chronic skin losses in patients with epidermolysis bullosa, a congenital blistering disorder.[52] Hefton et al. have employed this technology recently in treating chronic leg ulcers from a variety of causes.[53] Of the six wounds grafted, four were completely covered by full-thickness epidermis in 21–35 days after grafting, three of the four healed and remained covered for up to 2 years. The successful graft take was accompanied by rapid relief of pain. A comparable result was obtained in another study that we conducted with chronic leg ulcers.[54] The cultured autologous cell graft was done, in this instance, in two steps: first, the application of dermal fibroblast graft, followed by the epidermal cell graft. The best graft take was obtained in patients with chronic venous stasis ulcers. This new technology is promising and may be utilized in chronic cutaneous ulcers not amenable to other forms of treatment. More experience is needed, however, to improve the technology in this field.

REFERENCES

1. Krull E. A. (1985) *J. Am. Acad. Dermatol.* **12**, 394.
2. Friedman S. J. and Su W. P. D. (1983) *Am. Fam. Physician* **27**, 219.
3. Eaglstein W. H. (1985) *J. Am. Acad. Dermatol.* **12**, 434.
4. Winter G. D. (1962) *Nature* **193**, 293.
5. Winter G. D. and Scales J. T. (1963) *Nature* **197**, 91.
6. Hinman C. D. and Maibach H. I. (1963) *Nature* **197**, 377.
7. Rovee D. T., Kurowsky C. A., Labun J. et al. (1972) In: Maibach H. I. and Rovee D. T. (eds) *Epidermal Wound Healing*. Chicago, Year Book Medical Publishers, p. 159.
8. Winter G. D. (1977) In: Silver I. A., Erecinska M. and Bicher H. I. (eds) *Advances in Experimental Medicine and Biology*. New York, Plenum, p. 673.
9. Silver I. A. (1972) In: Maibach H. I. and Rovee D. T. (eds) *Epidermal Wound Healing*. Chicago, Year Book Medical Publishers, p. 291.
10. Hunt T. K. and Pai M. P. (1972) *Surg. Gynecol. Obstet.* **135**, 561.
11. Niinikoski J., Grislis G. and Hunt T. K. (1972) *Ann. Surg.* **175**, 588.
12. Balin A. K., Fisher A. J. and Carter D. M. (1984) *J. Exp. Med.* **160**, 152.
13. Banda M. J., Knighton D. R., Hunt T. K. et al. (1982) *Proc. Natl. Acad. Sci. USA* **79**, 7773.
14. Alvarez O. M., Metz P. M. and Eaglstein W. H. (1983) *J. Surg. Res.* **35**. 142.
15. Bennett R. G. (1982) Editorial. *J. Dermatol. Surg. Oncol.* **8**, 166.
16. Aly R. (1982) *Semin. Dermatol.* **1**, 137.
17. Mertz P. M., Marshall D. A. and Eaglstein W. H. (1985) *J. Am. Acad. Dermatol.* **12**, 662.
18. Varghese M. C., Balin A. K., Carter D. M. et al. (1986) *Arch. Dermatol.* **122**, 52.
19. Reed B. R. and Clark R. A. F. (1985) *J. Am. Acad. Dermatol.* **13**, 919.
20. Bartlet R. H. (1981) *J. Trauma* **21** (Suppl.), 731.
21. Alper J. C., Welch E. A., Ginsberg M. et al. (1983) *J. Am. Acad. Dermatol.* **8**, 347.
22. Braverman I. M., and Nasar M. A. (1981) *Practitioner* **225**, 1842.
23. Avakoff J. C. (1983) *Plast. Reconstr. Surg.* **72**, 576.
24. Angermeier M. C., Alper J. C. and Urbaniak H. S. (1984) *J. Dermatol. Surg. Oncol.* **10**, 384.
25. James J. H. and Watson A. C. H. (1975) *Br. J. Plast. Surg.* **28**, 107.
26. Caldwell F., Bowser B. H. and Crabtree J. H. (1981) *Ann. Surg.* **193**, 579.
27. Neal D. E., Whalley P. C., Flowers M. W. et al. (1981) *Br. J. Clin. Pract.* **35**, 254.
28. Turner T. D. (1985) In: Ryan T. J. (ed.) *An Environment for Healing: The Role of Occlusion. R. Soc. Med. Int. Cong. Symp. Ser.* **88**, 5.
29. Geronemus R. G. and Robins P. (1982) *J. Dermatol. Surg. Oncol.* **8**, 850.
30. Mandy S. H. (1983) *J. Dermatol. Surg. Oncol.* **9**, 153.
31. Tracy G. D., Lord R. S. A., Kibel C. et al. (1977) *Med. J. Aust.* **1**. 777.
32. Friedman S. J. and Su D. (1984) *Arch. Dermatol.* **120**, 1329.
33. Ryan T. J., Given H. F., Murphy J. J. et al. (1985) In: Ryan T. J. (ed.) *An Environment for Healing: The Role of Occlusion. R. Soc. Med. Int. Congr. Symp. Ser.* **88**, 99.
34. Groenewald J. H. (1985) In: Ryan T. J. (ed.) *An Environment for Healing: The Role of Occlusion. R. Soc. Med. Int. Congr. Symp. Ser.* **88**, 106.
35. Stevanovic D. V. (1985) In: Ryan T. J. (ed.) *An Environment for Healing: The Role of Occlusion. R. Soc. Med. Int. Congr. Symp. Ser.* **88**, 115.
36. Cherry G. W. and Ryan T. J. (1985) In: Ryan T. J. (ed.) *An Environment for Healing: The Role of Occlusion. R. Soc. Med. Int. Congr. Symp. Ser.* **88**, 61.
37. Jacobson S., Jonsson L., Rank F. et al. (1976) *Scand. J. Plast. Reconstr. Surg.* **10**, 97.
38. Pace W. E. (1978) *J. Dermatol. Surg. Oncol.* **4**, 678.
39. Romasz R. S., Barnhart M. D. and Schinagl E. F. (1978) *Angiology* **219**, 675.
40. Woodroof E. W. (1984) In: Wise D. (ed.) *Burn Wound Coverings*. Boca Raton, Fla, CRC Press Inc.

41. Hansbrough J. F., Zapata-Sirvent R., Carroll W. J. et al. (1984) *Burns* **10**, 415.
42. Warren R. J. and Snelling C. F. T. (1980) *Plast. Reconstr. Surg.* **66**, 361.
43. Nathan P., Macmillan B. G. and Holder I. A. (1974) *Appl. Microbiol.* **28**, 4665.
44. Shun A. and Ramsey-Stewart G. (1983) *Med. J. Aust.* **2**, 279.
45. Egan T. J., O'Driscoll J. and Thakar D. R. (1983) *Angiology* **1**, 197.
46. Faulk W. P., Matthews R., Stevens P. J. et al. (1980) *Lancet* **i**, 1156.
47. Robson M. C., Krizek T. J., Koss N. et al. (1973) *Surg. Gynecol. Obstet.* **136**, 904.
48. German J. C., Wooley T. E., Achauer B. et al. (1972) *Arch. Surg.* **104**, 800.
49. Aronoff M., Fleishman P. and Simon D. L. (1976) *J. Trauma* **16**, 280.
50. Eisinger M., Monden M., Raaf J.H. et al. (1980) *Surgery* **88**, 287.
51. Gallico G. G., O'Connor N. E., Compton C. C. et al. (1984) *N. Engl. J. Med.* **311**, 448.
52. Lin A. N., Balin A. K., Pratt L. et al. (1986) *J. Invest. Dermatol.* **186**, 489.
53. Hefton J. M., Caldwell D., Biozes D. G. et al. (1986) *J. Am. Acad. Dermatol.* **14**, 395.
54. Varghese M., Eisinger M. and Carter D. M. Unpublished.

Part III
TOPICS IN THERAPEUTICS

11. ADVERSE REACTIONS TO DRUGS IN THE ELDERLY

P. J. W. Scott

INTRODUCTION

Overall the elderly are more likely to suffer from adverse drug reactions (ADRs) than the young.[1] They are more likely to be admitted to hospital because of ADRs[2,3] and to suffer from ADRs while in hospital.[4] With many individual drugs they demonstrate an increased frequency of ADRs (e.g. flurazepam[5] and benoxaprofen[6]) but with others there is no significant change in ADRs with age (e.g. chlorpromazine[7] and propranolol[8]). The picture is further complicated as the incidence of different side-effects of the same drug may vary with age; the daytime sedation caused by nitrazepam increases with age, while nightmares do not.[9]

There is an increasing interest in the scientific basis of the susceptibility of the elderly to ADRs. However, to date the literature produced provides a somewhat patchy and erratic database. Reports of many ADRs are anecdotal and frequently the commonest, for example postural hypotension produced by prochlorperazine, seldom appear in literature. Furthermore studies that attempt to define the changes in drug disposition with age frequently rely on normal volunteers. This ignores the changes that may occur with disease, which are important when prescribing therapy for patients. On the other hand studies that examine hospitalized patients produce results that are also often misinterpreted when the effects of age *and* disease are confused with those of age *alone*.

Adverse drug reactions are reported in many different ways. In the UK perhaps the best known is the 'yellow card' system, which informs the Committee on the Safety of Medicines (CSM). Reporting of all ADRs with relevant clinical details is encouraged. As a result the CSM is able to produce regular reports concerning the incidence and severity of ADRs. Unfortunately as these summaries are mostly dependent on voluntary contributions they will therefore be incomplete. There is certainly a temptation to report interesting side-effects of new drugs, but how often do common ADRs to older drugs go unreported? It is unlikely, for instance, that the CSM would be able to give a balanced report on the incidence of allergic skin rashes to ampicillin. The blame for this lies with the medical profession who have become 'used to' such occurrences and fail to report them.

Another source of information are the results of surveys measuring the incidence of ADRs in the elderly. Williamson and Chopin reported that 12 per cent of elderly patients admitted to acute geriatric units in the UK were suffering from ADRs.[3] This type of study may exaggerate the occurrence of ADRs as the process of recording these events increases awareness, reduces the diagnostic threshold and may produce an artificially high incidence. The Boston Drug Surveillance Program has published many reports on the incidence of ADRs within a large number of hospital inpatients.[10] Once again such a survey may heighten the awareness to ADRs and produce a falsely high rate. Another criticism may be made when results are extrapolated from hospital patients to those living in the community. One of the best examples of such an error is seen in a study of serum albumin concentration in elderly inpatients.[11] Serum albumin is the most important binding protein for acidic drugs and in reduced concentration may increase the levels of free active drug predisposing to adverse effects (or increased therapeutic effect). This study demonstrated a reduction in serum albumin with age. A later study[12] did not confirm this finding. The original study had confused the effect of age *and* disease with the effect of age alone.

One of the commonest methods of recording ADRs is the 'case report'. This is being encouraged by the *British Medical Journal* whose editor will accept short unrefereed reports for rapid publication. Case reporting gives the opportunity for the author to demonstrate greater detail concerning the individual patient(s) than is possible in larger surveys. Also, information concerning rechallenge with the suspected drug can be given, which frequently gives additional proof to the ADR. For example, Price et al.[13] were able to give a report of hallucinations precipitated by ranitidine in a 72-year-old female. These disappeared with withdrawal of the drug and reappeared with its reintroduction. Such studies are very valuable but share the problem of the 'yellow card' reports in that an overall view of the importance and incidence of ADRs may be omitted.

ADRs are also reported within studies of therapeutic efficacy, for example of a new antihypertensive or non-steroidal anti-inflammatory agent. Such studies are essential prior to the release of a new drug or perhaps to the maintenance of its sales. There are generally two types of study design. First, the 'double blind' comparison with a placebo or another active drug and, second, the 'open' study. The blinded study tends to reduce doctor and patient bias but not to eliminate it. For example, it is virtually impossible to conduct a truly double blind study involving a beta-adrenergic antagonist as the lowering of the pulse rate identifies the type of drug being used. The problems with an open—or an incomplete—blinded study is that there is a tendency to exaggerate therapeutic efficacy, as it is 'obvious' that an antihypertensive agent 'must' lower blood pressure. This is not so. These studies may also tend to under-report ADRs as doctors subconsciously may not like to admit to their patients or themselves that their prescription has had a side-effect. In an open study of 1315 hypertensive patients receiving a combination of timolol and a diuretic the author reported an impressive response rate of almost 90 per cent with a 7 per cent incidence of adverse reactions.[14] These results have subsequently been used in the marketing of timolol, but the fact that the study was not blinded leaves unanswered significant questions concerning bias and therefore the overall relevance of the study.

Many studies of therapeutic efficacy involve too small a sample to comment authoritatively concerning the incidence or severity of ADRs. However, sometimes ADRs are so pronounced that trials have to be discontinued, as with a double blind comparison of baclofen compared with a placebo involving elderly stroke patients.[15] Drowsiness was so frequent that it led to the abandonment of the study.

DIAGNOSIS

The identification of ADRs in the elderly is not always easy. It may be virtually impossible to identify the drugs actually being taken. Probably the best way is to examine the drug containers, although labelling may be inadequate and the patient may have transferred drugs from their original containers.

Most ADRs occur within 2 weeks of starting therapy although some take longer, such as potassium depletion with diuretics or tardive dyskinesia with phenothiazines, which may occur many months after starting therapy. Not infrequently adverse reactions such as confusion or postural hypotension may be due to several drugs.

The diagnosis may be confirmed by improvement following withdrawal of the suspected drug although resolution of non-specific symptoms (for example confusion) may also be due to the treatment of a coincidental disease such as pneumonia. Rechallenging the patient with a suspected drug to demonstrate recurrence of symptoms is seldom carried out deliberately although it may happen by accident. ADRs with certain drugs (e.g. digoxin and anticonvulsants) may be identified by measurement of drug plasma concentration. The relationship between drug toxicity and plasma concentration is not always precise but it frequently provides a retrospective diagnosis of ADRs.

CAUSES OF SUSCEPTIBILITY OF THE ELDERLY TO ADRs

The causes of the age-related increase in ADRs are multiple but there is a direct correlation in the incidence with the number of drugs prescribed, for example,[16] from 5 per cent with 1 drug to 100 per cent with 10 drugs.

Compliance

Poor compliance is often blamed for ADRs but is more likely to offer protection, as drugs are usually omitted rather than taken in excess. However, difficulties can arise with confused patients who can mix up their drugs or take them too frequently. There have been several excellent reviews of compliance in the elderly.[17-19]

Pharmacokinetic Factors

Absorption of drugs from the gastrointestinal tract is little altered with increasing age. One interesting exception that may contribute to levodopa toxicity is the decline in gastric mucosal dopamine decarboxylase, which may be responsible for the considerably increased plasma levels of levodopa seen in the elderly.[20]

Presystemic elimination of drugs during their first pass through the liver in the portal system may be diminished by age. The first report of the disposition of propranolol in old age demonstrated a considerable increase in plasma concentration due to diminished first pass metabolism.[21] A subsequent report[22] failed to confirm this finding. The difference in the two studies appears to be that the former study involved patients and the latter normal volunteers. Therefore the change in the first pass metabolism of propranolol was due to disease rather than to age itself. This would suggest that the elderly sick would be at risk from propranolol toxicity but a survey of hospitalized patients receiving the drug failed to demonstrate a statistically significant increased incidence of ADRs.[8] The reasons for this lack of toxicity, despite high plasma levels, are complex. Perhaps the most important is that the dose of drugs such as propranolol is titrated against effect, avoiding overdosage. The protein binding of propranolol may also protect from adverse reactions. Propranolol is a basic drug and is principally bound to alpha-1-acid glycoprotein.[23] This is found in increased concentration in disease states.[24] The increased concentration of the inactive protein-bound propranolol would serve to protect the patient from ADRs. Finally there is a reduction in efficiency of the beta-1-adrenoceptor with increasing age,[25] which also might protect from adverse effects. Further support for this is seen in a study of hyperthyroid patients[26] in whom 160 mg/day of propranolol controlled symptoms at all ages without adverse effect, despite the elderly having higher plasma levels of the drug.

Albumin is quantitatively the most important plasma protein responsible for drug binding. Any lowering of plasma albumin would theoretically increase the unbound active drug concentration with increased potential for drug toxicity. Although albumin concentration is little changed in the fit elderly, it falls dramatically in the sick elderly. Clinically this results in an enhanced response to the drug or the development of toxicity at 'normal' total drug concentrations. This has been described for a number of drugs such as diazepam[27] and prednisolone.[28] Drug toxicity resulting from a reduction in albumin concentration is not always seen as the free drug is the fraction subject to metabolism and when protein binding is reduced the rate of metabolism may be increased, as with phenytoin.[29]

Once a drug has been absorbed, it will be distributed throughout the body depending on its physicochemical properties, for example whether it is fat- or water-soluble. This distribution of the drug may change with age as there is an increase in total body fat with an associated decrease in lean body mass.[30] Thus for fat-soluble drugs such as diazepam the volume of distribution increases with age.[31] The main importance of this is that fat-soluble drugs tend to have a longer elimination half-life with increasing patient age and this may contribute to the prolonged sedation caused by diazepam that is seen in the elderly.

Liver mass declines after the age of 50[32] and there is a direct relationship between liver mass and the efficiency of antipyrine metabolism.[33] This would suggest a reduction in the ability of the elderly liver to detoxify drugs, even though there appears to be no change in the concentration of at least five different enzymes involved in drug metabolism.[34] Reviewing the literature there is no evidence of an overall decline in drug metabolism with age; however, many of the studies are poorly designed and the calculations of rates of drug detoxification are inaccurate. This usually arises because experiments are conducted with oral administration of drugs. The assumption is made that bioavailability is 100 per cent, which may lead to considerable inaccuracies in subsequent calculations of clearance. To obtain definitive measurement of drug clearance (and of the volume of distribution) the drug has to be administered intravenously, ensuring 100 per cent bioavailability. In one study that examined the disposition of prazosin with age[35] both intravenous and oral dosing was used on separate study days. This revealed a 29 per cent reduction in bioavailability with age. There was also an increase in the plasma elimination half-life. Interestingly this prolongation of half-life was not due to a reduction in clearance but to an increase in the volume of distribution with age, which tends to reduce the drug plasma concentration and protects the patient from drug toxicity. If the prolongation of elimination half-life had been due to a reduction in the rate of clearance then accumulation and resultant toxicity might occur if the regular dose was not reduced.

An example of the problems that can arise when clearance is 'calculated' following oral administration may be seen in two studies concerned with the pharmacokinetics of atenolol with increasing age. In an 'oral-only' study the clearance of atenolol was shown to decline with age[36] while in a study that involved intravenous administration, no age-related change in clearance was noted.[37]

Adverse effects are more likely to be caused by the age-related decline in renal function[38] rather than by any decline in hepatic metabolism. There is substantial evidence for a fall with age in the rate of renal excretion of drugs such as kanamycin and gentamicin,[39] streptomycin and tetracycline,[40] cimetidine[41] and digoxin.[42] The potential for several of these drugs to cause toxicity (e.g. digoxin, gentamicin) is reduced by careful monitoring of plasma levels but in any case caution should be exercised when prescribing such drugs for the elderly.

Pharmacodynamic Factors

Drugs are considered to exert their action through specific receptors—a concept first proposed by Langley in 1878.[43] The effect of age on the sensitivity of drug receptors has recently been reviewed.[44] In many cases adverse reactions to drugs are caused by an exaggeration of the standard drug-receptor interaction, for example the day-time drowsiness caused by nitrazepam. Other adverse effects have no relationship to the therapeutic effect and in this case we must consider the presence of an *adverse* drug-receptor system, for example the haemolytic anaemia caused by methyldopa. The susceptibility of the elderly to ADRs might arise because of an alteration in the affinity and activity of drug receptors. While there is a limited amount of information available concerning changes in therapeutic receptors with age, there is virtually none concerning possible changes in adverse drug receptors.

There is no uniform rule that can be adopted concerning the effect of age on therapeutic drug-receptor sensitivity. The sensitivity to warfarin[45] and diazepam[46] increases with age, that to beta-adrenergic agonists decreases with age[24] while the sensitivity to alpha-adrenergic agonists remains unchanged.[47] The increase in receptor sensitivity to benzodiazepines is almost certainly responsible for the increase in toxicity demonstrated for flurazepam[5] and nitrazepam.[9] It is interesting that despite the shorter elimination half-life of temazepam when compared to nitrazepam, they both caused similar daytime sedation after seven night-time doses given to elderly patients.[48] The pharmacodynamic changes with age were more important than any kinetic differences.

The diminution in beta-adrenergic receptor efficiency with age may contribute to the lack of increase in toxicity with propranolol, despite higher plasma concentrations of the drug in the sick elderly.[8,21,26] There is little available information concerning the toxicity of alpha-adrenergic antagonists in the elderly.

PREVENTION OF ADRs IN THE ELDERLY

No drug will ever be entirely safe. Statutory drug regulation committees exist in most developed countries. Their function is to ensure that drugs on the market are monitored for safety and to screen new drugs prior to release. It is perhaps this latter duty that is the more difficult. All drugs have to complete a large number of safety checks, first in animals and then in volunteers, before obtaining a limited licence for administration to small groups of patients. In the past it has been considered unethical to conduct experiments on the elderly. Most study protocols excluded volunteers and patients over the age of 65. Apart from the 'ethical' objection difficulties were experienced in designing studies that recognized the multiple pathology present in many elderly patients.

The release of the non-steroidal anti-inflammatory agent benoxaprofen precipitated a crisis in drug regulation in the UK. Benoxaprofen completed the statutory safety examinations laid down at that time. The problem that rapidly became apparent arose because of inadequate testing in the elderly. It is possible that even a small study of elderly patients would have demonstrated significant ADRs. Halsey and Cardoe,[6] following the drug's release, demonstrated an 83 per cent incidence of ADRs in 42 patients over the age of 70. Sixty-nine per cent of these patients had to have therapy discontinued.

The World Health Organization published a paper entitled *The Control of Drugs for the Elderly* in 1981[49] in which many recommendations are made. These include proposals that all new drugs are evaluated and existing drugs reassessed to determine the effects in elderly subjects. They further recommend that physicians be educated to understand the problems of drug prescribing for the elderly and that the elderly themselves be better informed about the proper use of drugs. In the UK, drug regulations have been improved but problems remain. Drug companies have been instructed[50] to 'provide some positive, helpful advice to doctors on the use of the product in the elderly'. Data sheets were to be modified for inclusion in the 1985–86 Data Sheet Compendium[51] but there was no insistence on 'firm data'. A 'best estimate' of the factors that might affect drug response in the elderly was all that was required. For new drugs the position is more satisfactory. From 1 January 1985 all applications for the release of new drugs have to include clinical studies in the elderly where the drug is likely to be used in that age-group.

Unfortunately there are still major difficulties. Clinicians often learn of new drugs through pharmaceutical representatives. Results of studies are often represented in a simplified manner in advertisements with the attendant risk that vital information is omitted. In one advertisement (since withdrawn) the manufacturer of Madopar (benserazide/levodopa) demonstrated that their product was superior to another in improving the activities of daily living in a group of parkinsonian patients.[52] This was based on a study conducted by Admani et al.[53] Examination of this study demonstrates that with one exception there was no statistically significant difference between the two drugs. There was effectively no advantage of one drug over the other. The clinician must check original sources before accepting drug company advertising.

Another difficulty arises when considering the relevance of a particular study to drug safety. A pharmacokinetic examination of piroxicam, a non-steroidal anti-inflammatory drug (NSAID),[54] revealed that plasma concentration, elimination half-life and 'volume of distribution' (only oral dosing used) did not appear to be influenced by age or sex when compared with another study involving young adults. The conclusion was reached that elderly patients receiving the recommended dose of piroxicam were not exposed to undue risk due to any pharmacokinetic changes. In isolation this study might be misleading. One of the principal risks of prescribing NSAIDs is the risk of gastrointestinal ulceration, which is commonest in elderly females.[55] It is possible to calculate a risk ratio for NSAIDs based on the number of patients with associated peptic ulceration and the mean sales of these drugs in defined daily doses. In an example of such a calculation piroxicam had the greatest incidence of upper gastrointestinal ADRs when compared with indomethacin, naproxen, ibuprofen, fenprofen, diflunisal and ketoprofen.[56]

Weber and Griffin[57] from the Association of the British Pharmaceutical Industry have suggested that the elderly do not have an 'increase in overall susceptibility' to ADRs. They assert that a reduction in the number of adverse reactions experienced by the elderly might be achieved by avoidance of multiple therapy, greater care in the choice of medicines and more careful supervision of their use. Their advice is sound—the elderly are certainly liable to experience adverse drug interactions[58,59,60]—but the evidence from studies of benoxaprofen, benzodiazepines, anticoagulants and many others suggest that the elderly do indeed have an increased susceptibility to suffer from ADRs. It should be the acute concern of medical practitioners, the pharmaceutical industry and the statutory drug regulation committees to be aware of the problem and to find solutions.

Physicians must prescribe carefully and simply. They must review regularly prescriptions for elderly patients. They should certainly avoid prescribing drugs that the pharmaceutical industry claims can alleviate the process of ageing,[49] for example those drugs supposed to alleviate the consequences of declining cerebral function. These drugs have virtually no benefit; they only have side-effects.

The pharmaceutical industry must take its responsibility for the elderly very seriously indeed. The elderly consume 30 per cent of all NHS prescriptions[61] and deserve better protection than 'best estimates' would give.[50] Properly designed trials with elderly patients must be conducted with drugs that are liable to be used in this age-group. The results of these trials should be represented honestly and accurately in advertising material, which should be based on statistical analysis and not simply on opinion.

The drug regulation committees must remain aware of the particular sensitivity of the elderly to suffer ADRs and license drugs accordingly. Committees such as the CSM cannot function properly if there is an incomplete method of reporting ADRs. It is not sufficient to report only 'interesting' reactions but more common ones as well. Perhaps a more rapid and simplified method of reporting ADRs is desirable.

ADRs in the elderly are reaching epidemic proportions; we must all take responsibility to stem the tide.

REFERENCES

1. Caird F. I. and Scott P. J. W. (1986) *Drug-Induced Disorders. Vol. 2, Drug-induced Diseases in the Elderly: A Critical Survey of the Literature*. Amsterdam, New York, Oxford, Elsevier.
2. Levy M., Altwein W., Hillebrand J. et al. (1980) *Eur. J. Clin. Pharmacol.* **17**, 25.
3. Williamson J. and Chopin J. M. (1980) *Age Ageing* **9**, 73.
4. Hurwitz N. and Wade O. L. (1969) *Br. Med. J.* **1**, 531.
5. Greenblatt D. J., Allen M. D. and Shader R. I. (1977) *Clin. Pharmacol. Ther.* **21**, 355.
6. Halsey J. and Cardoe N. (1982) *Br. Med. J.* **284**, 1365.
7. Swett C. (1975) *Curr. Ther. Res.* **18**, 199.
8. Greenblatt D. J. and Koch-Weser J. (1973) *Am. Heart J.* **86**, 478.
9. Greenblatt D. J. and Allen M. D. (1978) *Br. J. Clin. Pharmacol.* **5**, 407.
10. Cohen M. R. (1974) *Hosp. Pharm.* **9**, 437.
11. Greenblatt D. J. (1979) *J. Am. Geriatr. Soc.* **27**, 20.
12. Hodkinson H. M. (ed.) (1984) *Clinical Biochemistry in the Elderly*. Edinburgh, Churchill Livingstone, p. 24.
13. Price W., Coli L., Brandstetter R. D. et al. (1985) *Eur. J. Clin. Pharmacol.* **29**, 375.
14. Head A. C. (1984) *Pharmatherapeutica* **3**, 650.
15. Hulme A., MacLennan W. J., Ritchie R. T. et al. (1985) *Eur. J. Clin. Pharmacol.* **29**, 467.
16. Kellway G. S. M. and McCrae E. (1973) *NZ Med. J.* **78**, 525.

17. Royal College of Physicians (1984) *J. R. Coll. Physicians Lond.* **18**, 7.
18. Denham M. 1984 In: Babagallo-Sangiorgi and Exton-Smith N. A. (ed.) *Ageing and Drug Therapy*. New York, Plenum Press.
19. Reid J. (1985) *J. Clin. Exp. Gerontol.* **7**, 31.
20. Warren P. M., Pepperman M. A. and Montgomery R. D. (1978) *Lancet* **ii**, 849.
21. Castleden C. M. and George C. F. (1979) *Br. J. Clin. Pharmacol.* **7**, 49.
22. Schneider R. E., Bishop H., Yates R. A. et al. (1980) *Br. J. Clin. Pharmacol.* **10**, 169.
23. Piafsky K. M., Borga O., Odar-Cederlof I. et al. (1978) *N. Engl. J. Med.* **299**, 1435.
24. Schneider R. E., Babb J., Bishop H. et al. (1976) *Br. Med. J.* **2**, 794.
25. Vestal R. E., Wood A. J. J. and Shand D. G. (1979) *Clin. Pharmacol. Ther.* **26**, 181.
26. Feely J. and Stevenson I. H. (1979) *J. Clin. Exp. Gerontol.* **1**, 173.
27. Greenblatt D. J. and Koch-Weser J. (1974) *Eur. J. Clin. Pharmacol.* **7**, 259.
28. Lewis G. P., Jusko W. J., Burke C. W. et al. (1971) *Lancet* **ii**, 778.
29. Hayes M. J., Langman M. J. S. and Short A. H. (1975) *Br. J. Clin. Pharmacol.* **2**, 73.
30. Novak L. P. (1972) *J. Gerontol.* **27**, 438.
31. Klotz U., Avant G. R., Hoyumpa A. et al. *J. Clin. Invest.* **55**, 347.
32. Thompson E. N. and Williams R. (1965) *Gut* **6**, 266.
33. Roberts C. J. C., Jackson L., Halliwell M. et al. (1976) *Br. J. Clin. Pharmacol.* **3**, 907.
34. Woodhouse K. W., Mutch E., Williams F. M. et al. (1984) *Age Ageing* **13**, 328.
35. Rubin P. C., Scott P. J. W. and Reid J. L. (1981) *Br. J. Clin. Pharmacol.* **12**, 401.
36. Rigby J. W., Scott A. K., Hawksworth G. M. et al. (1985) *Br. J. Clin. Pharmacol.* **20**, 327.
37. Rubin P. C., Scott P. J. W., McLean K. et al. (1982) *Br. J. Clin. Pharmacol.* **13**, 235.
38. Davies D. F. and Shock N. W. (1950) *J. Clin. Invest.* **29**, 496.
39. Lumholtz B., Kampmann J., Siersback-Neilsen K. et al. (1974) *Acta Med. Scand.* **196**, 521.
40. Vartia K. O. and Leikola E. (1960) *J. Gerontol.* **15**, 392.
41. Drayer D. E., Romankiewicz J., Lorenzo B. et al. (1982) *Clin. Pharmacol. Ther.* **31**, 45.
42. Roberts M. A. and Caird F. I. (1976) *Age Ageing* **5**, 214.
43. Langley J. N. (1878) *J. Physiol. Lond.* **1**, 339.
44. Scott P. J. W. (1982) *J. Clin. Exp. Gerontol.* **4**, 205.
45. Shepherd A. M. M., Hewick D. S., Moreland T. A. et al. (1977) *Br. J. Clin. Pharmacol.* **4**, 315.
46. Swift C. G., Ewen J. M., Clarke P. et al. (1985) *Br. J. Clin. Pharmacol.* **20**, 111.
47. Scott P. J. W. and Reid J. L. (1982) *Br. J. Clin. Pharmacol.* **13**, 237.
48. Cook P. J., Huggett A., Graham-Pole R. et al. (1983) *Br. Med. J.* **286**, 100.
49. World Health Organization (1981) Report on the Ninth European Symposium on Clinical Pharmacological Evaluation in Drug Control. *The Control of Drugs for the Elderly*. Copenhagen, World Health Organization.
50. Snell E. S. (1983) Letter from the Association of the British Pharmaceutical Industry to Member Companies.
51. Association of the British Pharmaceutical Industry (1985) *Data Sheet Compendium 1985–86*. London, Datapharm Publications Ltd.
52. Roche Pharmaceuticals. Advertisment: Parkinson's disease, P522261/385.
53. Admani A. K., Verma S., Cordingley G. J. et al. (1985) *Pharmatherapeutica* **4**, 132.
54. Darragh A., Gordon A. J., O'Byrne H. O. et al. (1985) *Eur. J. Clin. Pharmacol.* **28**, 305.
55. Walt R., Katschinski B., Logan R. et al. (1986) *Lancet* **i**, 489.
56. Collier D. St J. and Pain J. A. (1986) *Lancet* **i**, 971.
57. Weber J. C. P. and Griffin J. P. (1986) *Lancet* **i**, 1220.
58. Scott P. J. W., Stansfield J. and Williams B. O. (1982) *Health Bull.* **40**, 5.
59. Moir D. C. and Dingwall-Fordyce I. (1980) *J. Clin. Exp. Ther.* **4**, 329.
60. Gosney M. and Tallis R. (1984) *Lancet* **ii**, 564.
61. Crooks J. and Stevenson I. H. (1975) *Health Bull.* **33**, 222.

12. THE CHOICE OF ORAL HYPOGLYCAEMIC AGENT FOR THE ELDERLY

P. V. Knight

Approximately 1 in 10 of the population aged 65 years and over is diabetic.[1] Of these, in excess of 80 per cent will not require insulin therapy; but probably more than half of this group will be receiving an oral hypoglycaemic agent.[2] Currently the British National Formulary lists 11 such agents. Thus the practitioner is left with a wide and sometimes confusing choice. The ideal drug would be one that lowered blood glucose without producing hypoglycaemia or disrupting intermediary metabolism, had no appreciable side-effects and could be taken once a day. Unfortunately, such a drug is not yet in use.

INDICATIONS FOR ORAL HYPOGLYCAEMIC THERAPY

These should be no less stringent for elderly patients. What defines adequate diabetic control is, of course, a moot point that has long been debated. To allow elderly patients to continue with markedly elevated blood glucose levels is not a kindness, in the author's view. There is evidence that they will develop microvascular complications more rapidly than the young,[3] and they are certainly at risk of macrovascular disease and acute metabolic decompensation.[4]

It has been the author's practice to commence an oral agent if the postprandial blood glucose remains in excess of 12 mmol/l following one month of adequate dietary therapy. Oral agents should not be considered, by patient or physician, to be a substitute for diet.

WHICH DRUG?

Sulphonylureas

This group provides the majority of the agents currently available. They are all readily absorbed from the gastrointestinal tract and largely bound to plasma proteins. The drugs have a varying half-life, metabolism by the liver, and renal excretion. Their mode of action remains unclear even after 20 years of use. Currently, it is thought that sulphonylureas stimulate insulin secretion acutely,[5] but that their long-term hypoglycaemic action is related to a reduction of hepatic glucose release and to some effects around the insulin receptor site.[6,7]

Symptomatic hypoglycaemia may be produced by all the current agents, many of which also have a tendency to aggravate obesity. Chlorpropamide has a particularly long plasma half-life (*see Table* 12.1) and therefore may well produce prolonged nocturnal hypoglycaemia, which could be fatal in an elderly person.

Table 12.1. Oral hypoglycaemic drugs

Drug	*Plasma half-life (hr)*	*Daily dosage range (mg)*
Sulphonylureas		
Acetohexamide	1–3 (parent) 5 (metabolite)	250–1500
Chlorpropamide	35	100–500
Glibenclamide	10–16	2·5–15
Glibornuride	5–12	12·5–75
Gliclazide	10–12	40–320
Glipizide	3–7	2·5–30
Gliquidone	2–4	15–120
Glymidine	4	500–2000
Tolazamide	7	100–1000
Tolbutamide	7	500–2000
Biguanide		
Metformin	1–5	500–1500

Sources: *Martindale: The Extra Pharmacopoeia*, 28th ed., 1982
Association of the British Pharmaceutical Industry (1986) *Data Sheet Compendium 1986*. London, Datapharm Publications Ltd.

According to Bloom,[8] hypoglycaemia may occur for one of the following reasons:

1. The dose is too large in relation to the desired hypoglycaemic effect required and the patient's renal and hepatic function.
2. The patient may miss a meal, leading to hypoglycaemia, and this may be particularly problematical in patients with intellectual deficit.
3. As the sulphonylureas are highly protein bound, particularly those of the first generation, their hypoglycaemic effect may be enhanced by concomitant administration of drugs such as aspirin and warfarin.

Therefore, the rational choice of drug in a population who eat irregularly and may have diminished renal function is one that has a relatively short half-life, is extensively metabolized by the liver and has largely inactive metabolites, e.g. glipizide, gliquidone or gliclazide. Even these preparations are not perfect. Glipizide has been associated with nine hypoglycaemic episodes and gliclazide with four.[9] The first ever case of gliquidone associated with hypoglycaemia was recently reported[10] in a 73-year-old woman with marked renal failure. This emphasizes that all drugs are dangerous, especially in the elderly, and that their prescription should not be undertaken lightly. The last case quoted also demonstrates that oral hypoglycaemic therapy should be monitored at intervals and not simply forgotten about.

Since 1970, when the University Group Diabetes Program (UGDP) report was published,[11] there has been considerable controversy over the possible increased cardiovascular risk from sulphonylureas. In an elderly population, who may have established disease, this should be compared with the undoubted increased risk from uncontrolled diabetes.

Metformin

Metformin is the only biguanide currently available in the UK. It does not produce symptomatic hypoglycaemia and may also have a useful weight-reducing effect.[12,13]

There are three main theories to its mechanism of action:

1. Inhibition of intestinal glucose absorption.
2. Increased peripheral utilization of glucose.
3. Inhibition of hepatic glucose production.

The drug may be used either alone or in combination with a sulphonylurea.[14]

Metformin's major drawback is the disruption of intermediary metabolism,[15] in particular the production of fatal lactic acidosis. Thus it has been suggested that metformin should be avoided in cases of cardiac, renal, respiratory and hepatic dysfunction.[13,15] Random age barriers of 60, 65 and 75 years have also been quoted.[11,15,16] Knight et al.[17] have suggested that an arbitrary age barrier is not justified, as an increase in plasma lactate (a measure of intermediary metabolism) is not associated with age *per se*. It was argued that metformin might be prescribed in the elderly, provided renal function was within normal limits (for the elderly) and the patient did not exhibit overt cardiac, respiratory or hepatic failure.

It is unfair to visit the sins of phenformin on metformin, as there was not a single case of metformin-induced lactic acidosis in the UK between 1972 and 1982.[18] All the incidents quoted by Assan et al.[19] occurred in the presence of acute renal failure.

Guar Gum

Guar is not strictly an oral hypoglycaemic, but has been shown in some studies to decrease postprandial blood glucose.[20] However, a recent study of elderly diabetics failed to substantiate this, but did show a significant decrease in body weight.[21]

CONCLUSION

A decision to commence oral hypoglycaemic therapy should be taken only when adequate dietary restriction has failed. A careful assessment of the patient's cardiorespiratory status should be made, in conjunction with estimates of renal and hepatic function.

It is best to begin with a short-acting sulphonylurea such as gliquidone, especially if the patient is near normal weight. Should the patient be markedly obese, then metformin is useful, either alone or as an adjunct to sulphonylurea therapy, provided it is prescribed—as with all drugs in the elderly—after careful deliberation.

REFERENCES

1. Mehnert H., Sewering H., Reichstein W. et al. (1968) *Dtsch. Med. Wochenschr.* **93**, 2044.
2. Gatling W., Houston A. C. and Hill R. D. (1985) *J. R. Coll. Physicians Lond.* **19**, 248.
3. Caird F. I., Pirie A. and Ramsell T. G. (1969) *Diabetes and the Eye*. Oxford and Edinburgh, Blackwell Scientific.
4. Pirart J. (1978) *Diabetes Care* **1**, 168.
5. Barnes A. J., Garbieu K. J. T., Crowley M. F. et al. (1975) *Lancet* **ii**, 69.
6. Kolterman O. G., Prince M. J. and Olefsky J. M. (1983) *Am. J. Med.* **74**. 102.
7. Lockwood D. H., Maloff B. L., Nowak S. M. et al. (1983) *Am. J. Med.* **74**, 102.
8. Bloom A. (1977) *Clin. Endocrinol. Metab.* **6**, 499.
9. Campbell I. W. (1985) *Horm. Metab. Res. (Suppl.)* **15**, 105.
10. Hamilton D. A. and Campbell I. W. (1986) *Pract. Diabetes* **3**, 261.
11. University Group Diabetes Program (1970) *Diabetes* **19**, 789.
12. Clarke B. F. and Duncan L. J. P. (1968) *Lancet* **i**, 123.
13. Herman L. S. (1979) *Diabete Metab.* **3**, 233.
14. Clarke B. F. and Duncan L. J. P. (1965) *Lancet* **i**, 1248.
15. Luft D., Schmulling R. M. and Eggstein M. (1978) *Diabetologia* **14**, 75.
16. Berger W. (1979) *Pharmakritik* **1**, 9.
17. Knight P. V., Semple C. S. and Kesson C. M. (1986) *J. Clin. Exp. Gerontol.* **8**, 51.
18. Campbell I. W. (1984) *Br. Med. J.* **289**:, 289.
19. Assan R., Heuelin C., Geneval D. et al. (1977) *Diabetologia* **13**, 211.
20. Jenkins D. J. A., Goff D. V., Leeds A. R. et al. (1976) *Lancet* **ii**, 172.
21. Canning G. Personal Communication.

13. THE MANAGEMENT OF HYPOTHERMIA

W.J. MacLennan

The rational management of hypothermia is dependent on a clear understanding of both the causes and complications of the condition.

AETIOLOGY

Ill health may cause hypothermia by interfering with an individual's inability to feel cold, or to respond appropriately to a cold environment. Again it may interfere with the complex regulatory mechanism designed to maintain body temperature.

Among the most common neurological conditions responsible for hypothermia are cerebrovascular disease and Parkinsonism where hypothalamic damage and restricted mobility combine to interfere with thermoregulation.[1] In dementia due to senile dementia of Alzheimer's type or multiple cerebral infarcts there are the further problems that patients may be unable to appreciate a change in temperature or respond to it in an appropriate fashion. Added to the problems of neurological disease is the fact that most old people have impaired autonomic function so that they show an inadequate vasoconstrictor response to cold.[2,3]

Under normal cicumstances the thyroid gland plays little part in the temperature regulation of humans, but thyroid hormone depletion in myxoedema is a classic cause of hypothermia.[4] Diabetic patients are also at increased risk of hypothermia either because of an autonomic neuropathy, or, more commonly, because of impaired glucose utilization in ketoacidosis.[5] At the opposite end of the scale hypoglycaemia due to insulin or sulphonylurea excess may also cause hypothermia.[6]

A further problem frequently linked with hypothermia is subnutrition associated with emaciation.[7] It has been suggested that the problem here is one of inadequate thermogenesis due to reduced stores of brown fat. However, the current view is that humans have inadequate supplies of the lipid for it to play an important part in temperature regulation.[8] Some other explanation for the link between subnutrition and hypothermia must be sought.

Among patients admitted to hospital with hypothermia, the most common finding is that an acute illness has overwhelmed temperature regulation.[9] This may be a pneumonia, peritonitis, septicaemia, uraemia, electrolyte imbalance or congestive cardiac failure, and in this situation it is often the severity of the underlying illness rather than the hypothermia that is responsible for an adverse prognosis.[10]

Major tranquillizers and tricyclic antidepressants have a potent effect on hypothalamic and autonomic function and significantly increase the risk of hypothermia in elderly patients.[11] Benzodiazepine hypnotics are less likely to cause problems, but even these have occasionally been implicated in hypothermia.[12,13]

Alcoholism is increasingly being recognized as a problem in the elderly and often occurs in the most unexpected situations.[14] Peripheral vasodilatation, a resetting of the hypothalamic thermostat, and an inappropriate response to cold all conspire to increase the incidence of hypothermia.[15]

COMPLICATIONS

Hypothermia causes a wide range of organic disorders and, in clinical practice, it can be extremely difficult to distinguish these from the multiple pathology that is often responsible for the condition. An example is that almost every patient with hypothermia has a bronchopneumonia.[1] This is easily missed since a reduced body temperature may slow both pulse and respiratory rates, and a reduced tidal volume makes respiratory sounds inaudible.

A large proportion of patients develop atrial fibrillation, and at a temperature of less than 30 °C there is a particularly high risk of ventricular fibrillation.[16] Manoeuvres such as endotracheal intubation, cardiac catheterization, external rewarming or even lifting the patient on and off a stretcher may be enough to induce this.[17]

In all patients the blood pressure is low as is the cardiac output, but these are often adequate to meet the reduced metabolic needs of hypothermic organs. Problems tend to arise when injudicious rewarming causes peripheral vasodilatation. The cardiac output is then inadequate to meet the needs of the increased vascular pool, and severe shock ensues.

An increased capillary permeability allows plasma protein to leak into the extravascular compartment with the result that there is a rise in the blood haematocrit and viscosity.[18] This often leads to diffuse intravascular coagulation with thrombotic and haemorrhagic lesions throughout the body.[19] Clinical manifestations of these include myocardial infarction, stroke, renal tubular necrosis, mesenteric infarction and gastrointestinal haemorrhage.

One of the most common complications of diffuse intravascular coagulation is acute pancreatitis.[20] In hypothermia the clinical signs of this are minimal, and the diagnosis is made on the basis of abnormal serum biochemistry.

INVESTIGATION

Patients with hypothermia should have a full clinical assessment, but the nature of the condition is such that it often masks the signs and symptoms of both its causes and complications. Adequate laboratory investigation, therefore, is particularly important. It should be recognized, however, that the myocardium is in a parlous state so care should be exercised even in performing a venepuncture or in taking the patient on and off a radiology table.

Interpretation of haematological results is difficult in that haemoconcentration may conceal the effects of a gastrointestinal haemorrhage, or that hypothermia suppresses a white cell response to infection. A blood film showing schistocytes and a low platelet count provides useful confirmation of diffuse intravascular coagulation.

Even in the absence of renal tubular necrosis, a reduced cardiac output, haemoconcentration and the effects of ageing on renal function invariably produce increases in blood urea and creatinine concentrations. Reduced metabolic activity means that evidence of renal damage may only become apparent as the body temperature rises. It is important, therefore, to monitor blood and urinary biochemistry and urinary output for several days after the episode.

Interpretation of blood gas values is confounded by the problem that rewarming prior to analysis causes a fall in the pH and a rise in the Po_2 and Pco_2, so that specially designed nomograms are required to correct for this.[21] Obviously it is essential that the laboratory be given information on the core temperature of the patient.

After correction for temperature the pH is usually low, the Po_2 low and the Pco_2 high.[18] Factors contributing to this pattern include respiratory failure with carbon dioxide retention, hypovolaemia with metabolic acidosis, and, in the earlier phase of the illness, lactic acidosis due to shivering.

Blood glucose levels are usually elevated as a result of decreased tissue utilization and pancreatic damage with a reduction in insulin secretion.[22,23] Changes in glucose levels and acid base balance due to hypothermia should be distinguished from diabetic ketoacidosis causing hypothermia. Distinguishing features include a previous history of diabetes and the severity of the hyperglaecaemia. The latter requires active treatment with insulin and fluid and electrolyte replacement, whereas the hyperglaecaemia of hypothermia often resolves as the body temperature returns to normal.[23]

Despite the formidable reputation of acute pancreatitis there is little association between serum amylase levels and mortality from hypothermia.[20] However, a proportion of patients with pancreatitis go on to develop diabetic ketoacidosis a few days after the resolution of hypothermia and serum amylase levels are useful in identifying this at-risk group.

Thyroid function tests should be performed to identify the subgroup of patients in whom hypothermia is due to hypothyroidism. Hypothermia and the disorders causing and associated with it may modify the serum thyroxine level so that it is essential to confirm the diagnosis by checking for an elevation of the serum thyroid stimulating hormone concentration.[24] Unfortunately, there is an inevitable delay in performing thyroid function tests, so that clinicians are faced with the much more difficult task of making an immediate diagnosis on the basis of a history and clinical signs.

Changes in myocardial and skeletal muscle permeability produce increased concentrations of serum creatinine phosphokinase and lactic dehydrogenase.[25] They are therefore of no diagnostic value in identifying cardiac or muscle necrosis, but merely cause difficulty and are best not measured.

Stress and impaired corticosteroid utilization result in elevated serum cortisol levels.[26] Clinicians who have gone to the length of measuring cortisol levels after the administration of tetracosactrin (Synacthen) have found an impaired response. This is the result of a deranged adrenal metabolism, however, and corrects itself after the patient is rewarmed.

An electrocardiograph usually shows a J wave deflection at the junction of the QRS complex and the ST segment, a feature pathognomonic of hypothermia.[27] Other changes include lengthening of the PR and QT intervals and inversion of the T waves. These characteristics are mainly of academic interest and the principal reason for performing an electrocardiogram is to identify a myocardial infarction causing or resulting from the hypothermia. The changes may only become apparent after the patient is rewarmed so that a repeat tracing should be performed at this stage if there is any doubt.

A chest X-ray film usually confirms the presence of a bronchopneumonia. It may also identify some pulmonary oedema resulting from a change in capillary permeability, but this often resolves without diuretic therapy being given as the condition of the patient improves.[28]

Patients with severe hypothermia may be pulseless. In these circumstances the condition also suppresses electroencephalographic activity.[29] Thus, a flat tracing does not necessarily indicate brain death and an attempt at resuscitation should normally be made.

TREATMENT

Rapid Rewarming

A variety of dramatic measures can be taken to correct the body temperature of a hypothermic patient rapidly. The principle behind these is that an attempt is made to warm the central body core rather than the cutaneous periphery. Rapid rewarming of the limbs inevitably causes peripheral vasodilatation with diversion of blood from the brain and kidneys with severe and usually fatal circulatory collapse.

The least invasive of these techniques is to apply radiant heat to the torso taking the temperature up to 35 °C, and thereafter allowing it to rise spontaneously.[30] Internal rewarming may also be achieved by administering warm fluids by a nasogastric or rectal tube.[31]

A more heroic measure is to open the thorax and bathe the anterior mediastinum in warm saline.[32] Even in an elderly person this may be a reasonable approach if he or she has developed ventricular fibrillation. At temperatures below 30 °C this is usually unresponsive to countershock. Mediastinal irrigation combined with open cardiac massage may keep the patient alive for long enough for defibrillation to be attempted at a higher core temperature.

Other means of rapidly infusing warm fluids are peritoneal dialysis, haemodialysis or an arteriovenous shunt connected to a heat exchanger and oxygenator.[18,33,34] Finally air rather than fluid can be used in the rewarming medium.[35] This can be done by inserting an endotracheal tube and using a ventilator linked to a heated humidifier to instil air at 40 °C.

A major objection to most of these methods is that they involve a considerable amount of instrumentation that may well trigger off a fatal cardiac arrhythmia in hypothermic patients. There is the further consideration that hypothermia may protect a patient against the adverse effects of a disturbed metabolism. Rapid rewarming often results in the metabolic demands of organs outpacing an impaired homeostasis. Careful monitoring and correction of abnormalities are essential, but frequently ineffective. Finally there is the ethical consideration that the parlous condition of the patient may be the result of an irreversible disorder causing the hypothermia. In such circumstances energetic intervention may be inappropriate.

Gradual Rewarming

The prerequisite for this approach is patience.[28] Treatment takes place in a room with a temperature between 20° and 30 °C. Heat loss is prevented by using one or, at most, two blankets. The rectal temperature should be monitored and if the rise in this exceeds 0.5 °C in an hour, rewarming should be slowed down by taking away the blankets. A foil blanket produces more rapid rewarming but often causes circulatory collapse,[36] and should not be used under any circumstances.

There has been considerable debate about the relative merits of rapid as against gradual rewarming.[36] This has not been resolved in that proponents of the two methods treated different types of patients. There is no firm evidence, however, that in elderly patients rapid rewarming achieves a lower mortality. Under these circumstances there would seem to be merit in adopting the simpler approach.

Supportive Measures

The range of causes and complications of hypothermia is such that there is a strong argument for managing all cases in an intensive care unit.

Since most patients have bronchopneumonia, and many also have pulmonary congestion, all should be given oxygen. This should be delivered at 28 per cent through a face mask. Endotracheal intubation often triggers off ventricular fibrillation in hypothermia and should only be used in exceptional circumstances. Antibiotics also are mandatory and should be given parenterally. Either amoxycillin or co-trimoxazole is acceptable in most cases.

A fine clinical judgement is required in deciding whether or not to use parenteral fluids. Increased capillary permeability means that even dehydrated patients with hypothermia may have a high skin turgor, and whereas all patients show some increase in blood urea levels only a proportion require fluid replacement. An exception is hypothermia due to diabetic ketoacidosis where large quantities of fluid are required. The effects of age, disease and cold on cardiac function mean that patients run a fine balance between dehydration and fluid overload. Bearing in mind the dangers of increased cardiac irritability it is probably best to avoid a central venous pressure line and to monitor the situation clinically.

There are several measures that should *not* be taken in hypothermia. An example is that the acidosis associated with the condition resolves spontaneously as the temperature returns to normal. Parenteral bicarbonate is of no value in this situation. An exception is acidosis due to diabetic ketoacidosis. Again, since there is no evidence that there is adrenal insufficiency in hypothermia there is no reason why clinicians should give corticosteroids.

Patients who have hypothermia due to myxoedema should be given 20 μg of tri-iodothyronine parenterally. However, the preparation is of no value in euthyroid patients, and increases the risk of death from a cardiac arrhythmia.[37] The problems of diagnosing myxoedema in hypothermia have already been emphasized. If there is doubt it may be reasonable to wait until the hypothermia has resolved, and the clinical signs can be more precisely defined before resorting to supplements.[1]

The cardiac complications of hypothermia require particularly careful treatment. Those patients who have atrial flutter or fibrillation should only receive digoxin if it fails to resolve on rewarming. Clinical evidence of pulmonary oedema is an indication for intravenous frusemide.

If a patient presents with ventricular asystole or fibrillation it is important to recognize that hypothermia protects the brain against the metabolic effects of cardiac arrest and that prolonged survival is possible.[38,39] Standard countershock techniques should be applied if the core temperature is above 30 °C. Below this level the heart is refractory to countershock, so that mediastinal perfusion and open heart massage are necessary.

If the patient is successfully rewarmed, other complications such as stroke, renal medullary necrosis or mesenteric infarction manifest themselves and require appropriate treatment. It is also at this stage that the condition causing the hypothermia often becomes obvious necessitating a radical reappraisal of management.

Hypothermia is perhaps best considered as an episode in a continuum of disease. Rewarming and supportive measures are simple and relatively safe as long as the clinician is patient. However, the cause of the hypothermia often carries a poor prognosis, while the complications after rewarming often fully exercise the resources of an intensive care unit.

REFERENCES

1. Fitzgerald F. R. and Jessop C. (1982) *Adv. Intern. Med.* **27**, 127.
2. Collins K. J., Exton-Smith A. N., James M. H. et al. (1980) *Age Ageing* **9**, 17.
3. MacLennan W. J., Hall M. R. P. and Timothy J. I. (1980) *Age Ageing* **9**, 25.
4. Forester C. F. (1963) *Arch. Intern. Med.* **111**, 734.
5. Gale E. M., Tattersall R. B. (1978) *Br. Med. J.* **2**, 1387.
6. Stranch B. S., Felig P., Baxter J. D. et al. (1969) *JAMA* **210**, 345.
7. Bastow M. D., Rawling J. and Allinson S. P. (1983) *Lancet* **i**, 143.
8. Hervey G. R. and Tobin G. (1983) *Clin. Sci.* **64**, 7.
9. Whittle J. L. and Bates J. H. (1979) *Arch. Intern. Med.* **139**, 418.
10. Bryant R. E., Hood A. F., Hood C. E. et al. (1971) *Arch. Intern. Med.* **127**, 120.
11. Korczyn A. D. (1980) In: Dukes M. N. G. (ed.) *Meyer's Side Effects of Drugs.* Amsterdam, Excerpta Medica, p. 76.
12. Impallomani M. and Ezyat R. (1977) *Br. Med. J.* **i**, 223.
13. Naylor G. J. and McHarg A. (1977) *Br. Med. J.* **ii**, 22.
14. Post F. (1982) In: Levy R. and Post F. (eds) *The Psychiatry of Late Life.* London, Blackwell, p. 180.
15. Lomax P., Bojarek J. G., Chesarck W. A. et al. (1980) *Pharmacology* **21**, 288.
16. Towne W. D., Geiss W. P. and Yanes H. O. (1972) *N. Engl. J. Med.* **287**, 1135.
17. Southwick F. S. and Dalglish P. H. (1980) *JAMA* **243**, 1250.
18. Reuler J. B. (1978) *Ann. Intern. Med.* **89**, 519.
19. Duguid H., Simpson R. G. and Stowers J. M. (1961) *Lancet* **ii**, 1213.
20. Maclean D., Murison J. and Griffiths P. D. (1973) *Br. Med. J.* **4**, 757.
21. Kelman G. R. and Nunn J. F. (1966) *J. Appl. Physiol.* **21**, 1484.
22. Fuhrman G. J. and Fuhrman F. A. (1963) *Am. J. Physiol.* **205**, 181.
23. Stoner H. B., Frayn K. N., Little R. A. et al. (1980) *Clin. Sci.* **59**, 19.
24. Thomson J. A. (1980) In: Exton-Smith A. N. and Caird F. I. (1980) *Metabolic and Nutritional Disorders in the Elderly.* Bristol, John Wright, p. 199.
25. Carlson C. J., Emilson B. and Rapaport E. (1978) *Am. Heart J.* **95**, 352.
26. Felicetta J. V., Green W. L. and Goodner C. J. (1980) *J. Clin. Endocrinol. Metab.* **50**, 93.

27. Emslie-Smith D. (1958) *Lancet* **ii**, 492.
28. Emslie-Smith D. (1981) *Br. J. Hosp. Med.* **26**, 442.
29. Martyn J. W. (1981) *Can. Med. Assoc. J.* **125**, 1089.
30. Ledingham I. M. and Mone J. G. (1980) *Br. Med. J.* **i**, 1102.
31. Bristow G., Smith R. and Lee J. (1977) *Can. Med. Assoc. J.* **177**, 242.
32. Coughlin F. (1973) *N. Engl. J. Med.* **288**, 326.
33. Pickering B. G., Bristow G. K. and Craig D. B. (1977) *Anesth. Analg.* **56**, 574.
34. Lee H. A. and Ames A. C. (1965) *Br. Med. J.* **i**, 1217.
35. Shanks C. A. and Marsh H. M. (1973) *Br. J. Anaesth.* **45**, 522.
36. Maclean D. and Emslie-Smith D. (1977) *Accidental Hypothermia.* Oxford, Blackwell.
37. Hylander B. and Rosenquist V. (1985) *Acta Endocrinol.* **108**, 65.
38. Althaus V., Aebeshard P. and Schupbach P. (1982) *Ann. Surg.* **195**, 492.
39. Nordrchaugh J. E. (1982) *Br. Med. J.* **i**, 867.

Part IV
FUTURE DEVELOPMENTS

14. FUTURE DEVELOPMENTS IN GERIATRIC MEDICINE

R. E. Irvine

It is said that one can only be sure of two things in the future, death and taxes. But we can be sure also that there will be an expanding role for geriatric medicine.

DEMOGRAPHY

Table 14.1 shows the demographic changes (actual and expected) between 1951 and 2021. The clientele of geriatric medicine is broadly the population over the age of 75. The biggest growth in their numbers has already taken place—1·3 million between 1951 and 1981. There will be a further 1·1 million extra between 1981 and 2021; two-thirds of that increase will have taken place by 1991. It is already nearly over, and the heavens have not fallen.

Table 14.1. Elderly population (in millions) in England and Wales, 1951–2021

	Age group (years)			
Year	*65–74*	*75–84*	*85+*	*Total 75+*
1951	3·2	1·4	0·2	1·6
1981	4·6	2·4	0·5	2·9
1991	4·5	2·8	0·8	3·6
2001	4·2	2·8	1·0	3·8
2011	4·5	2·6	1·1	3·7
2021	5·1	2·9	1·1	4·0

Source: Annual Abstract of Statistics (1986) and Craig J. (1983) *Population Trends No. 3*. London, Office of Population Censuses and Surveys.

There will be an extra half-million over-85s by the end of this century and 20 per cent of them may need residential care, but to double their numbers will only increase their proportion in the population from 1 to 2 per cent. In Hastings where the author spent his working life the proportion was 3 per cent. The local community had no difficulty in adapting to their needs. They were a valuable source of employment. *Figure* 14.1 is also reassuring. It shows that the proportion of active workers to pensioners will show little change over the next 25 years.[1]

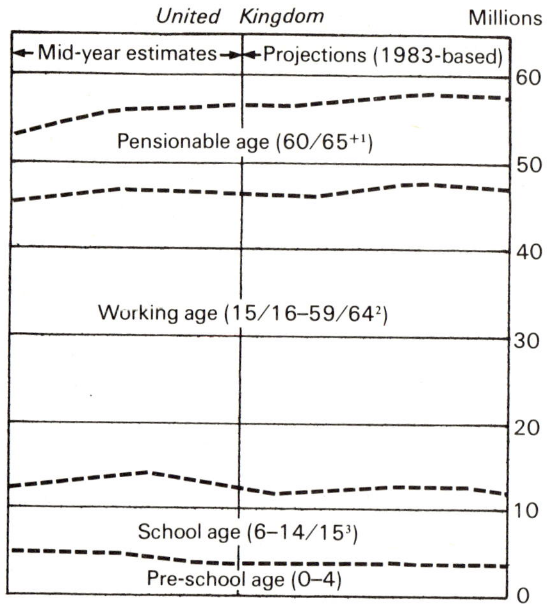

Fig. 14.1 Population by age-groups.

[1] 60 for females, 65 for males.
[2] 59 for females, 64 for males.
[3] School-leaving age raised to 16 in 1972.
Source: Office of Population Censuses and Surveys; Government Actuary's Department.
Reproduced by courtesy of the Controller of HMSO.

PREVENTION OF DISEASE

We now have the knowledge to prevent many of the diseases of late life. We often fail to do so, but we know how to prevent cancer of the lung, stroke, ischaemic heart disease and much of diabetes. Today's non-smokers, joggers and weight-watchers may well enjoy a healthier old age.

NEED FOR SERVICES

We know that all forms of illness, both physical and mental, become commoner as age advances and that the elderly are the biggest consumers of health and social services. Expenditure per head on those aged 75 and over is 2·5 times that spent on those aged 65–74, and 4·5 times that spent on the population generally.[2]

Apart from Parkinsonism neurological disorders still defeat us, nor do we know how to prevent the degenerative diseases of later life such as osteoarthritis, cataracts, hernia and prostatic hypertrophy, but surgical skill can correct many of these conditions—a marvellous way to turn the clock back. And the pacemaker is a modern miracle. These life-enhancing miracles have one inescapable side-effect: everything that prolongs life increases the risk of ultimate dementia, perhaps the greatest challenge of our time to geriatric medicine and to the health and social services generally. When technology has so much to offer it is not surprising that the number of people over 75 going into hospital increased by 20 per cent between 1970 and 1983. Most went to the surgical specialties, psychiatry and general medicine. Less than one-third went to geriatric medicine.[3,4]

GROWTH OF GERIATRIC MEDICINE

Nevertheless geriatric medicine continues to expand. A decade ago there was doubt whether it could survive.[5] But the specialty is evidently alive and well,[6] and recruitment is now excellent.[7] In 1985 the Royal College of Physicians established the Diploma in Geriatric Medicine, and in 1984 it awarded the prestigious Moxon medal for clinical research to a geriatrician, Professor Norman Exton-Smith.

Table 14.2. Hospital discharges and deaths in England, 1979 and 1983

Specialty	*1979*	*1983*
General medicine	808 854	836 606
Paediatrics	276 280	313 058
Geriatric medicine	258 819	324 634
Nine medical specialties*	248 478	259 343

* Cardiology, diseases of the chest, dermatology, genito-urinary medicine, infectious diseases, neurology, rehabilitation, rheumatology, young disabled.
Source: Department of Health and Social Security/Office of Population Censuses and Surveys, Hospital In-Patient Enquiry 1979 and *1983*. London, HMSO.

In 1983 for the first time more patients were discharged from geriatric wards than from paediatric ones, making geriatrics after general medicine the second largest medical specialty in terms of the number of inpatients treated.[4] *Table* 14.2 shows how discharges from geriatric wards now outnumber those from all medical specialties combined, apart from general medicine. Indeed only general medicine, general surgery, orthopaedics and gynaecology discharged more patients, making geriatric medicine the fifth largest specialty in the NHS.[4]

In terms of consultant numbers geriatric medicine with 487 consultants is 10th out of 50 specialties and is growing faster than any other. New posts are being created at a rate of 15–20 per year.[8] We shall not reach the Department of Health and Social Security's target of 800 consultant posts by 1990,[9] but within a decade geriatrics may well have become the second largest specialty in medicine.

AN ACUTE SPECIALTY

Official terminology still contrasts geriatric medicine with the acute specialties, and it is true that our responsibilities include the provision of continuing care. But the fact is that geriatric medicine is becoming an ever more acute specialty, and this trend is likely to continue. In 1972 the average length of stay in geriatric wards was 105 days. In 1983 it was 52 days; in Hastings the figure was 31. The median duration of stay, the time by which half the patients admitted have been discharged, was 16 days in 1983.[4] It will soon be less than 2 weeks.

The principles of acute geriatric medicine were first taught by Olbrich and Woodford-Williams in Sunderland in the 1950s and were rediscovered by Hodkinson and Jefferys at Northwick Park nearly 20 years later.[10] It has been suggested that an emphasis on acute geriatric medicine will lead once again to neglect of the patients whose needs originally justified our specialty and who are now in our rehabilitation and long-stay wards.[6,11] I do not believe this to be true. An acute service takes all-comers and must neglect no one of appropriate age. Teamwork, concern for carers and built-in rehabilitation are all equally relevant. As the whole history of geriatric medicine shows, an acute approach reduces the need for long-stay care, returns more people to the community in better shape and reassures their carers.

GERIATRIC MEDICINE AND THE DISTRICT GENERAL HOSPITAL

An acute geriatric service cannot function without beds in the main district general hospital (DGH). Access to the full range of diagnostic facilities is essential. Many old people need a great deal of investigation. Because of the non-specific presentation of disease in old age many tests are done routinely. The future will see an increased demand for all forms of investigation, which will make the need for beds in the DGH even more pressing than it is today.

How Many Beds in the DGH?

How many beds will be required? The present answer given by the Department of Health and Social Security is 'a sufficient number'. Norms have been abandoned. But until 5 years ago the policy was to suggest that 3 beds per 1000 over 65 would be sufficient for acute purposes, with a further 2 per 1000 over 65 for rehabilitation 'preferably in the DGH but otherwise in a general hospital with other acute beds and appropriate facilities'. Up to 5 more beds were suggested for continuing care.[9] In Hastings, which has exceptional private facilities, there were 1·8 beds per 1000 for acute geriatric medicine, and 2·5 beds 'with appropriate facilities' for rehabilitation, including geriatric orthopaedics. These beds were sufficient to run an acute service for many years without a waiting list, suggesting that the 1981 norms were about right. In terms of the population over 75 the bed ratios were 3·9 for acute medicine and 5·7 for rehabilitation; in round numbers 10 beds per 1000 in this age-group require the facilities of the DGH.

GERIATRIC MEDICINE AND GENERAL MEDICINE

The Department of Health and Social Security norms are essentially empirical. They have been criticized by Grimley Evans, who claims with good reason that in a world in which 40 per cent of medical patients over the age of 75 go to general medicine and only 60 per cent to geriatric medicine, services to the elderly cannot be properly assessed unless the joint contributions of general and geriatric medicine are considered together.[11]

From a study of the published results of some successful geriatric services Grimley Evans[12] suggests that an effective service depends on the availability of 9 beds per 1000 over 65 with DGH facilities from the combined resources of both the general and geriatric medical departments. Grimley Evans' famous table has been adapted in *Table* 14.3 to include the figures for Hastings in 1984. Admittedly some of his data are 15 years old but the comparison may still perhaps be of some interest. Hastings, as part of the so-called 'Costa Geriatrica', has always been a generation ahead of the rest of the country in terms of the age structure of its inhabitants. In 1985 it had a population of 161 800 of whom 26 per cent were over 65, 12·5 per cent over 75 and 3 per cent over 85.

Hastings and Other Services

Hastings has managed for many years on a considerably smaller allocation of geriatric beds than the successful services quoted by Grimley Evans. With 6·9 beds per 1000 over 65 it is well below the national average of 8·6 (*see Table* 14.3). With 4·3 beds per 1000 over 65 having DGH facilities, Hastings has fewer such beds than the successful services but even so is almost 50 per cent better off than the national average of 2·8.

Hastings has more general medical beds available to the elderly than two out of the three successful services, but at 1·4 beds per 1000 over

Table 14.3. Beds per 1000 persons aged 65 and over in Hastings compared with four successful geriatric services

	Hull (1974)	*Oldham (1972)*	*Sunderland (1971)*	*West Newcastle (1981)*	*England and Wales (1971–1974)*	*Hastings (1983)*
A All geriatric beds	8·1	9·1	9·0	7·6	8·6	6·9
B Geriatric beds with DGH facilities	5·7	8·5	8·5	2·0	2·8	4·3
C Other DGH medical beds for elderly	3·0	0·5	1·0	3·9	2·6	1·4
D All beds for elderly (A + C)	11·1	9·6	10·0	11·3	11·2	8·3
E All DGH beds for elderly (B + C)	8·7	9·0	9·5	5·9	5·4	5·7
G Annual medical admission rate	120	60	82	80	76	101

Sources: Evans J. Grimley (1983) *Community Med.* **5**, 242; South East Thames Regional Health Authority (1986) *Regional Information Profile 1984*. Bexhill, SETRHA.

65 is about 50 per cent below the national average and a long way below West Newcastle, which has almost three times as many (3·9 per 1000).

The total number of beds available for the elderly (combined geriatric and general medical resources) is, at 8·3, well below the national figure of 11·2 and below the successful services, which are all close to the national average (*see Table* 14.3).

And in the total number of available beds with DGH facilities for the elderly Hastings is far below Grimley Evans' suggested figure of 9 beds per 1000 over 65. With 5·7 beds per 1000 Hastings is barely above the national average of 5·4; 2·5 per 1000 of these beds are used for rehabilitation (*see above*).

The figure for Hastings for annual medical admissions per 1000 over 65 is greater than in any service except Hull. Perhaps this reflects the high risk of hospitalization in a population with an exceptional number of very old people.

General Practitioner Beds

All geriatric services depend on local factors. *Table* 14.3 does not include 45 general practitioner beds (1·1 per 1000 over 65), which almost exclusively serve the elderly. Almost two-thirds have access to diagnostic facilities but, of course, there are no junior staff.[13]

Community Services

The community health and social services have always worked well in Hastings and Bexhill, although the home help and meals on wheels services are less than one-third those in London.[13] The quality of general practice is high and the selection of patients for referral excellent.

Psychiatry

Hastings has a first-class psychogeriatric service created by Dr T. Venkateswarlu. There is an eight-bedded joint psychogeriatric assessment ward in the same block as the acute geriatric wards. The availability of immediate psychiatric help is a priceless asset.

The Private Sector

There are a large number of private nursing homes in Hastings, 36 homes with 955 beds in 1984, a number that is still growing.[13] There are also over 2000 places in residential homes in the area, so that it is seldom difficult to discharge a patient who is ready to move on. The private sector helps the NHS to improve turnover. It creates confidence that patients will not get stuck in hospital. Anyone can be accepted. There is no need for any defensiveness or for routine domiciliary assessment.

PATTERNS OF PRACTICE

It is no longer necessary to argue, as we once had to, that beds in the district general hospital are a necessity for an effective service. The original chronic sick model is obsolete and unacceptable. All geriatric services must be able to take acutely ill patients. There is, however, still room for debate about the pattern of practice. There are three acceptable models.

Selective Service

A selective service takes those patients judged suitable for it by the local general practitioners. These are usually the infirm elderly with multiple medical and social problems and non-specific presentation.[14] Routine domiciliary visiting is often a feature of the service. The selective pattern is probably still the most common; several fine academic departments are built on this model. Their weakness perhaps lies in the identification of geriatric medicine too much with decrepit old age rather than with old age generally, and they thus risk perpetuating the clinical undertaker image of the geriatrician.[15]

Age-defined Service

The age-defined service, established in Hull by Horrocks,[16] takes unselected emergencies over a certain age, often 75 (in Hastings 76) and sometimes as high as 80 years. Admission is direct, often in the daytime through a secretary in the departmental office, giving a single point of referral and a prompt response to a doctor who wants to get a patient admitted. Domiciliary visiting is confined to non-urgent patients and plays a small part in such a service.

The workload of the physician is very high. In Hastings in 1984 two geriatricians admitted the same number of emergencies as four general physicians,[13] and in 1985 considerably more. Although the work is hard the job satisfaction is enormous.

Integrated Service

In an integrated service there is no separate acute geriatric ward. All patients, whatever their age, go to common acute medical wards run by a firm of physicians. One physician has special responsibility for the elderly (PSRE). He or she has a general medical take-day like the other physicians, and is responsible for giving geriatric advice to colleagues and for providing rehabilitation and long-stay facilities for those patients who require them. The emergency workload of the PSRE is less because, except on the take-day, the physician's colleagues are responsible for the elderly patients.[17]

Variations

Mixed arrangements are possible. For example, an age-defined policy can be operated in respect of patients from the accident department only, or on certain days of the week, or between certain hours. An age-defined policy may be agreed for patients under 65 and over 75 while a selective policy is applied to those aged between 65 and 75.

In an integrated system less urgent patients may go direct to the rehabilitation wards. In Oxford, which is well endowed with physicians, patients are admitted to a common acute ward but referring doctors can specify whether they would like their patients of any age admitted under a general physician or a PSRE.[18]

WHICH PATTERN FOR THE FUTURE?

Each system has its advantages and disadvantages. Both the selective and the integrated systems are established in professorial departments. I do not know of a pure age-related service in a teaching hospital, and this policy has been specifically eschewed in Scotland.[19]

We can be certain of one thing. No one system will be right for everybody. There are various interests to be considered.

Patients and Carers

As far as patients and their carers are concerned we have no data, but the author would suspect that the age-defined service is more beneficial. The patient enters an environment designed for his or her welfare and is sure of a welcome. The patient's carers, too, will perhaps be better understood by a staff specially attuned to their needs. In an age-defined service there will be a lot of coming and going. Patients may find that their fears of being in a geriatric ward are groundless. A selective ward risks having the opposite effect because all patients are by definition very infirm. More than once in the Department of Medicine for the Elderly in Hastings the author was told 'Thank God my mother is not in a geriatric ward'. In a mixed ward, even an integrated one run with the best intentions, an older person is at risk of taking second place to younger patients who may be perceived as more urgent or interesting. And is death so normal and well managed?

Doctors

The new patterns of practice evolved because of dissatisfaction with the selective system. They represent efforts to find a more positive identity for geriatric medicine.

Both are popular with the doctors who work in them. In Hastings the author and his colleagues found that the age-related system gave intense job satisfaction to all the staff, and two recent surveys among senior registrars showed a preference for purely geriatric work.[20,21]

Those running integrated services are equally enthusiastic.[18] Three years ago advertisements for PSREs were reported to attract more applications than any other jobs in geriatric medicine.[22] The author knows of one doctor who inherited an age-defined service but changed to an integrated one because it allowed more time for the rehabilitation and long-stay wards. The integrated pattern ensures that general wards are adapted to the elderly and promotes collaboration between the physicians, but tensions may arise if the pool of beds is inadequate.

Although doubts have been expressed,[23] the policy of expanding the specialty has certainly been correct and the greatest need is still for more consultants. In the author's view they should be trained in both general and geriatric medicine even if they eventually work full time in geriatrics. Their value as physicians is enhanced if they can offer a special investigative skill. The author knows of one PSRE who is also colonoscopist to his London teaching hospital; we need more like him.

Efficiency

The proponents of both age-defined and integrated services claim to make better use of beds. Either system will lead to an improved turnover. The integrated system is claimed to be more efficient on the grounds that no one is turned away from a geriatric ward when a medical bed is empty. But this need not happen in an age-defined service either if, as in Hastings, a spirit of give and take exists among the physicians with a readiness to lend and borrow beds. An age-related policy is only possible when there are sufficient geriatric beds with access to the facilities of the district general hospital, about 5 beds per 1000 over 65 (10 per 1000 over 75). The integrated pattern is better when there is a good allocation of general medical beds but few geriatric beds in the DGH.

We need information about the cost effectiveness of the various models. In the absence of convincing evidence to show the superiority of one system over another, the future development of geriatric medicine will be pragmatic. Different patterns will develop in different places as a result of different circumstances, but the move towards a more acute service will maintain its momentum.

CONTINUING CARE

With an increasing trend to short-stay, high-turnover activity in departments of geriatric medicine, what will happen to those who need continuing care?

Continuing Care Outside the National Health Service

Caird reminds us that geriatrics began in the long-stay chronic sick wards and that geriatricians are still identified by the public and by colleagues as long-stay doctors.[24] We have only recently become aware of the amount of care that is now provided outside the NHS by the voluntary and private sectors. In England the private sector is about twice as big as the voluntary. There are no figures to distinguish the two in Scotland and Wales.[25]

Table 14.4. Long-stay nursing care in England and Wales, 1984

	No. of persons	*% Long-stay beds*
NHS geriatric beds	34 200	44·5
NHS psychiatric beds	19 900	25·9
Private/voluntary nursing homes	22 800	29·6
Total	76 900	100·00

Source: Laing W. (1985) *Private Health Care.* London, Office of Health Economics.

Table 14.4 shows that just over half the elderly who are receiving continuing care in England and Wales are not under physicians in geriatric medicine; one-quarter are in mental hospitals and rather more in private and voluntary nursing homes. There are marked national variations. In England 30 per cent are cared for outside the NHS, in Wales 23 per cent, but in Scotland only 11 per cent. Yet even in Scotland only two-thirds are the responsibility of geriatric medicine.[25,26]

A similar situation exists in the field of residential care. In England almost half of all residential care is provided outside the public sector and in Scotland and Wales over one-third.[25,26]

The Rise of Private Care

Figure 14.2 taken from the work of William Laing for the Office of Health Economics, shows the changes in various forms of continuing

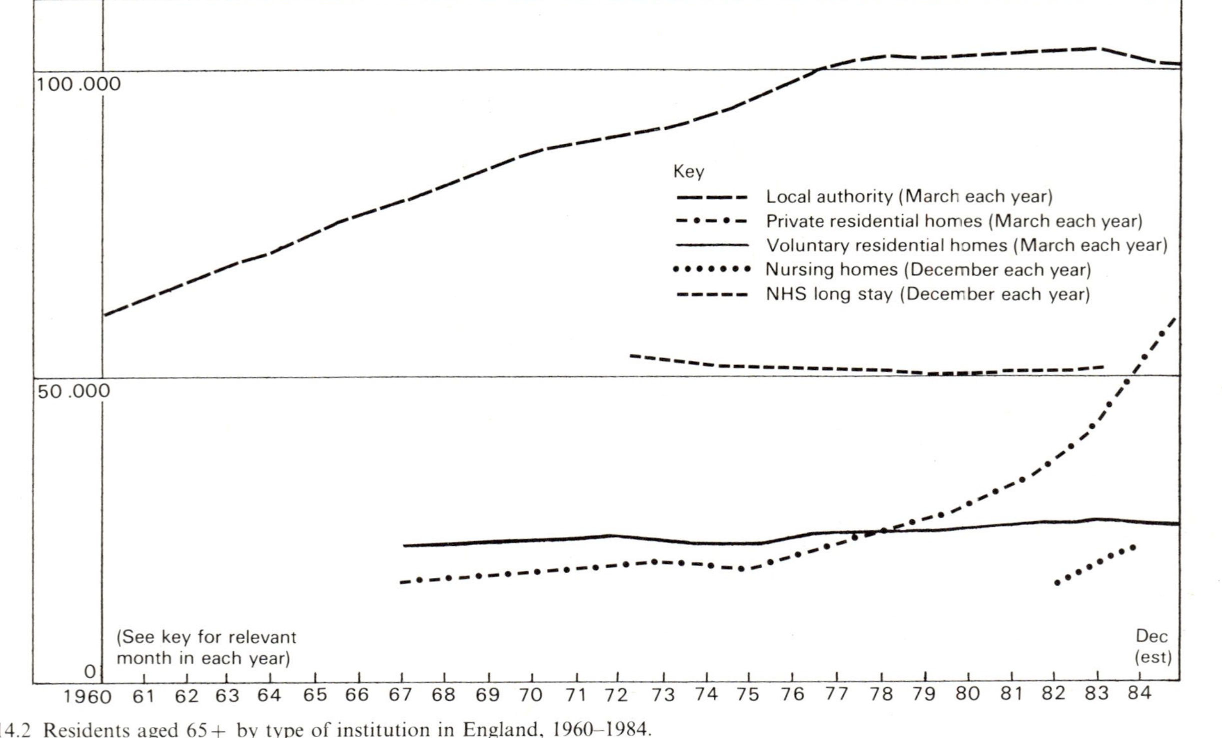

Fig. 14.2 Residents aged 65+ by type of institution in England, 1960–1984.

Sources: DHSS Residential Accommodation Statistics for local authority provided and registered residential accommodation, with estimates for December 1984 based on local authority registrations.
SBH 212 returns for nursing homes, adjusted for bed occupancy and estimated for 1984 on the basis of health authority registrations.
Reproduced by courtesy of the Office of Health Economics.

care, including residential homes and nursing homes, since 1960. During this time the population over the age of 75 has grown from 2·0 to 3·5 million. Geriatric long-stay beds have declined by 5000 since 1974, but this has been offset by a matching increase in beds with DGH facilities, which is very welcome.

Local authority provision grew steadily during the early years of the Welfare State but peaked in 1977. Since then it has not increased, though substandard accommodation continues to be replaced gradually.

Voluntary homes also show little change, but private residential homes show a spectacular increase that has accelerated since 1982. This sector has quadrupled in the past 20 years. Reliable figures for nursing homes did not exist before 1982 but they too have grown by one-third in the past 3 years.[25]

Can the growth of the private sector continue to meet the demand for residential and nursing home care? One may hope that it will. Only two things are likely to kill the goose that is laying the golden egg: one is impossibly high standards, the other is inadequate supplementary benefit (SB). If standards are set too high then homes will go out of business. It is in the interest of the registration authorities, the NHS and the social services, who are unable to provide the care themselves, to help these homes to keep going. Between 30 and 40 per cent of residents are funded by SB payments, and if these are set at too low a level then homes will avoid taking people who are dependent on SB. But these are matters for negotiation.

There is unlikely to be a political threat to private homes, provided standards are maintained; a recent national survey on this point was reassuring.[27] A government that cannot provide the necessary care in the public sector would be unwise to drive out those who can. It is good news also that the British Geriatrics Society is having talks with the Registered Nursing Homes Association, whose members are concerned about standards and value for money.

Value for Money

There is little doubt that private care costs less. The average cost in a long-stay geriatric hospital in 1983–1984 was £243 per week. In Hastings in 1984–1985 it was £291, 10 per cent lower than the regional average. NHS costs include drugs, dressings, medical salaries, remedial therapy and chiropody, which would figure in the costs of a private nursing home, but they exclude the cost of the buildings. Except in its experimental NHS nursing homes the NHS cannot offer the privacy of a single room.

In the private sector the average charge in 1984 was £166, which includes the cost of the buildings. Using 1982–1983 prices Wright estimated that there was a difference of 33 per cent between a contractual bed in a nursing home and one in an NHS long-stay ward.[28] Using figures from 1983–1984 Capewell et al. in Edinburgh found differences of a similar order.[29] The private sector appears to be able to provide long-stay nursing care for two-thirds of what it costs the NHS and can often offer privacy into the bargain.

Comparing Like with Like

But this is only true if like is compared with like. Is it certain that patients in long-stay geriatric wards and in private nursing homes are comparable in their need for nursing care? One study found higher dependency in the private sector[30] but most have found that nursing home patients are less dependent than those in NHS long-stay wards.[28,29,31] Wright made a financial adjustment for the lower dependency of nursing home patients but even so found that private care gave better value than the NHS.[28]

Continuing Care in the NHS

It seems likely, therefore, that an increasing amount of continuing care will be taken over by the private sector. This will be to the advantage of the geriatric service since it should release resources for what the NHS does better than anyone—acute geriatric medicine and rehabilitation.

But the NHS must retain some share in the provision of continuing care. A department of geriatric medicine needs beds, perhaps about 50 in a district, for the care of the most difficult patients, those with behavioural disorders and those with exceptional physical problems such as extreme obesity, extreme helplessness and feeding difficulties. A continuing care unit is also an excellent place for respite care provided the patient's condition is stable.

Continuing care facilities are needed for research and training, particularly nursing training, and for the credibility of geriatric medicine generally. Professor Millard's new unit at Bolingbroke Hospital in the St George's Hospital group is a marvellous example of what can be achieved under the NHS.

Organization of Continuing Care

There are many unsolved problems in the provision of continuing care and debate will continue. The most certain thing in the author's view is that the physician in geriatric medicine, advised by a multi-disciplinary team, should control the entry to NHS-funded long-term care. Beds are our crucial resource. Geriatricians are the only clinicians with an overall view. We are the experts in using beds to the best advantage. It is the oldest principle of geriatrics that no one should enter long-term care without proper assessment. The best way to ensure this is to provide an efficient acute geriatric service. The aim is to make it easier for general practitioners with patients who cannot stay at home to get their patients admitted to hospital than to seek any alternative solution. It is then certain that the patients will receive full multidisciplinary assessment before any decisions are made about long-term care, whether in the private or the public sector.

Once such patients enter long-term care, however, it is much less certain whether it is necessary for geriatricians to retain responsibility for day-to-day management. There are others who can do this, for example clinical assistants or the patient's own general practitioner. In Hastings as many patients went to private nursing homes under their own doctors as to our own continuing care beds. The author is unaware that they suffered by escaping from consultant care.

NHS Nursing Homes

An attempt to provide continuing care within the NHS without involving the consultant in day-to-day care can be seen in the experimental NHS nursing home, of which there are three in England. They are the subject of a multidisciplinary research project that will compare the patients' care and quality of life with those provided in a conventional long-stay ward. A report is expected in 1988.[32]

Patients are only accepted after full geriatric assessment but once admitted they return to the care of their own doctors. As in a private nursing home the nurse, not the consultant, is in overall charge. Standards are higher than in the NHS wards. Single rooms are the norm. Costs may be higher than in a conventional long-stay ward and these, as we have seen earlier, are more expensive than in a private nursing home.

The crucial factor affecting the future of these homes is likely to be economic. Under the NHS patients receive continuing care free, irrespective of income, but in local authority residential care they are assessed financially and pay according to their means. It seems unlikely that the NHS with all its burdens will invest much in this type of care when a similar service can be provided in the private sector without cost to the NHS. It would seem more sensible to introduce nursing care into local authority homes; this is to be attempted in Hastings though the experiment has not yet started.

Collaboration

The public and the private sectors are interdependent. The statutory responsibility for the registration of homes gives each a continuous interest in the other. Practical collaboration consists first and foremost in referring patients and their relatives to suitable homes. It is one of the primary responsibilities of social workers in a geriatric team to know the local homes and to select the right patients for them. It is disgraceful when relatives are simply handed a list of addresses and left to get on with it. The decision to abolish the old-fashioned medical social worker was a disaster. In the author's view it is quite likely that the NHS will be forced to employ social workers of its own if it wishes to ensure an effective geriatric service.

There may also be an opportunity for collaboration in physiotherapy and occupational therapy. Therapy is not regularly available in many homes, and it would be appropriate for community-based therapists to visit private homes if requested, not so much to treat individual patients as to give advice and encouragement to the staff. Patients from nursing homes who need rehabilitation should be welcome to come to the day hospital for treatment.

COMMUNITY SERVICES

Geriatric medicine has shown its worth to society by its ability to assist in situations that were formerly regarded as hopeless, by its provision of immediate help to old people who in times past might have been denied admission to hospital, and by its willingness to take all comers from its catchment area.

But the ability to do this depends on the knowledge that we can get people out of hospital as well as into it. For a few this depends on places in nursing homes or residential homes, whether public or private. But for many it depends on the availability of community health and social services to support the elderly person's carers or to substitute for them when necessary. Like hospitals the community services are under pressure.

There is no space here to go into these issues, which are of vital importance. Anyone concerned is recommended to read the British Medical Association's excellent new report *All Our Tomorrows.*[2] It suggests that too often we take advantage of the goodwill of individual carers and that in many places community services are inadequate.

Perhaps it is partly a matter of organization. In Hastings the primary care teams were excellent and some of the ablest social workers were the home help organizers. I cannot remember a time when we had to keep a patient in hospital who was ready to go home because home help could not be arranged. And most carers achieve marvels provided their needs are considered as well as those of the patient, and the right help is offered at the right time.

CONCLUSION

The demographic pressures of the next 50 years ensure a great future for geriatric medicine. We shall respond to these pressures by treating more people for less time in a more acute model of care.

The form in which geriatric services are organized to achieve this, whether selective, age-defined or integrated, will be a matter for decision locally. The vital common factor is sufficient beds in the district general hospital.

Wider recognition of the rewards and opportunities in geriatric medicine will produce excellent recruits. It is important that they are trained in general medicine as well as in geriatric medicine and that they are competent in some form of investigative technology.

Continuing care will be provided on an increasing scale by sources that do not depend on NHS funds. The private sector is growing. We need to collaborate with it and to welcome it, but we should not abandon all continuing care within the NHS. We need it for training, for research and for our own credibility.

All our efforts could be undermined unless community services keep pace with what can be achieved in hospital.

ACKNOWLEDGEMENTS

I am grateful to the Editor of *Social Trends* and to the Director of the Office of Health Economics for permission to reproduce *Figs*. 14.1 and 14.2.

I am grateful also for information and advice to Dr Norman Melia of the Department of Health and Social Security; Mr A. R. Martindale CB, General Manager of Hastings Health Authority; Mrs Anne Taylor, Librarian, Hastings Postgraduate Centre; the Hastings physicians; and Dr T. M. Strouthidis and my erstwhile colleagues of all disciplines in the Department of Medicine for the Elderly in Hastings.

REFERENCES

1. *Social Trends* (1986) **16**, 22. London, HMSO.
2. British Medical Association (1986) *All Our Tomorrows: Growing old in Britain*. London, BMA.
3. Department of Health and Social Security/Office of Population Censuses and Surveys (1979) *Hospital In-Patient Enquiry 1979*. London, HMSO.
4. Department of Health and Social Security/Office of Population Censuses and Surveys (1983) *Hospital In-Patient Enquiry 1983*. London, HMSO.
5. Leonard J. C. (1976) *Br. Med. J.* **ii**, 1335.
6. Coni N. (1985) *Health Policy* **5**, 173.
7. Barker W. H. and Williamson J. (1986) *Br. Med. J.* **293**, 896.
8. Department of Health and Social Security (1984) *Health Trends* **17**, 45.

9. Department of Health and Social Security (1981) *The Respective Roles of the General Acute and Geriatric Sectors in the Care of the Elderly Hospital In-Patient.* London, HMSO.
10. Hodkinson M. and Jefferys P. M. (1972) *Br. Med. J.* **iv**, 536.
11. Stout R. W. and Moffatt W. H. (1984) *Geriatr. Med.* **14**, 136.
12. Evans J. Grimley (1983) *Community Med.* **5**, 242.
13. South East Thames Regional Health Authority (1986) *Regional Information Profile 1984.* Bexhill, SETRHA.
14. Brocklehurst J. C. (1985) In: Brocklehurst J. C. (ed.) *Geriatric Medicine and Gerontology*, 3rd ed. Edinburgh, Churchill Livingstone.
15. Adams G. F. (1964) *Lancet* **i**, 1055.
16. Horrocks P. (1982) In: Isaacs B. (ed.) *Recent Advances in Geriatric Medicine 2.* Edinburgh, Churchill Livingstone.
17. Evans J. Grimley (1983) *Lancet* **i**, 1430.
18. Evans J. Grimley and Graham J. M. (1984) *J. R. Coll. Physicians Lond.* **18**, 18.
19. Bouchier I. A. and Williamson J. (1982) *Health Bull.* **40**, 179.
20. Donaldson M. (1985) *Age Ageing* **14**, 8.
21. Knight P. V. (1986) *J. R. Coll. Physicians Lond.* **20**, 271.
22. Graham J. M. and Playfair H. R. (1983) *Health Trends* **15**, 66.
23. Batchelor Sir I. (1984) *Policies for a Crisis.* London, Nuffield Provincial Hospitals Trust.
24. Caird F. I. (1982) In: Caird F. I. and Evans J. Grimley (eds) *Advanced Geriatric Medicine 2.* London, Pitman.
25. Laing W. (1985) *Private Health Care.* London, Office of Health Economics.
26. Primrose W. R. and Capewell A. E. (1986) *Health Bull.* **44**, 81.
27. Day P. and Klein R. (1985) *Br. Med. J.* **290**, 1020.
28. Wright K. (1985) *Public Money* June, 52.
29. Capewell A. E., Primrose W. R. and MacIntyre C. (1986) *Br. Med. J.* **292**, 1719.
30. Bennett J. (1986) *Br. Med. J.* **293**, 867.
31. McMahon D. G., Bhakri H. L. and Bowman C. F. (1986) *Br. Med. J.* **293**, 265.
32. Graham J. M. (1983) *Age Ageing* **12**, 273.

Index